Eye and Vision Research Developments

Modern Data about Age-Related Cataract Pathogenesis in Humans

EYE AND VISION RESEARCH DEVELOPMENTS

Additional books in this series can be found on Nova's website under the Series tab.

Additional e-books in this series can be found on Nova's website under the e-book tab.

EYE AND VISION RESEARCH DEVELOPMENTS

MODERN DATA ABOUT AGE-RELATED CATARACT PATHOGENESIS IN HUMANS

N. V. KORSAKOVA

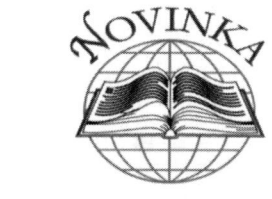

Nova Science Publishers, Inc.
New York

Copyright © 2012 by Nova Science Publishers, Inc.

All rights reserved. No part of this book may be reproduced, stored in a retrieval system or transmitted in any form or by any means: electronic, electrostatic, magnetic, tape, mechanical photocopying, recording or otherwise without the written permission of the Publisher.

For permission to use material from this book please contact us:
Telephone 631-231-7269; Fax 631-231-8175
Web Site: http://www.novapublishers.com

NOTICE TO THE READER

The Publisher has taken reasonable care in the preparation of this book, but makes no expressed or implied warranty of any kind and assumes no responsibility for any errors or omissions. No liability is assumed for incidental or consequential damages in connection with or arising out of information contained in this book. The Publisher shall not be liable for any special, consequential, or exemplary damages resulting, in whole or in part, from the readers' use of, or reliance upon, this material. Any parts of this book based on government reports are so indicated and copyright is claimed for those parts to the extent applicable to compilations of such works.

Independent verification should be sought for any data, advice or recommendations contained in this book. In addition, no responsibility is assumed by the publisher for any injury and/or damage to persons or property arising from any methods, products, instructions, ideas or otherwise contained in this publication.

This publication is designed to provide accurate and authoritative information with regard to the subject matter covered herein. It is sold with the clear understanding that the Publisher is not engaged in rendering legal or any other professional services. If legal or any other expert assistance is required, the services of a competent person should be sought. FROM A DECLARATION OF PARTICIPANTS JOINTLY ADOPTED BY A COMMITTEE OF THE AMERICAN BAR ASSOCIATION AND A COMMITTEE OF PUBLISHERS.

Additional color graphics may be available in the e-book version of this book.

Library of Congress Cataloging-in-Publication Data

Library of Congress Control Number: 2012937538

ISBN: 978-1-62081-823-7

Published by Nova Science Publishers, Inc. † New York

Contents

Abstract		vii
Introduction		ix
Chapter I	Development, Structure and Regeneration of the Lens	1
Chapter II	The Human Lens Normally and in Age Cataract Formation	9
Chapter III	Biogenic Amines Role in the Functioning of Eye's Tissues	21
Chapter IV	Material and Methods	27
Chapter V	Results	31
Chapter VI	Results' Discussion	39
Conclusion		47
Appendix		49
References		59
Index		77

Abstract

The given book deals with one of the most actual problem of modern medicine – the establishment of humoral factors' role in age cataract pathogenesis of a human being. Fundamental distinctions of neuromediator supply of the processes of different kinds of formations of age cataract, first described in the given monograph, are the evidence of different pathogenic mechanisms, determining the character of age neurodystrophic process proceeding in the human lens. The aim of this monograph is to attract attention of investigators to the pathogenically proved necessity of differentiated approach of formation of preventive and therapeutic measures of human age cataract depending on its specific kind.

Conclusions: This book discovered the significant differences in morphological and immunohistochemical status of lens cells in age-related cortical and nuclear cataract forming. This demonstrates the necessity of the differentiated view formation to study the pathogenesis of age-related cataract in human depended on its type.

Audience: histologists, physiologists, ophthalmologists, gerontologists, post-graduates and senior students of higher medical learning institutions.

Introduction

Today, the significant increase of age cataract morbidity is marked out all over the world [24]; it has been referred to as the main cause of blindness in the world [122] and considered as the "medico-social problem of national importance" [59, 109].

According to data of G. Venkataswamy et al. (1989) [190], the primary signs of age cataract are revealed in 64-68% patients over 60, and practically all people suffer from age cataract after 80.

In the world, there number about 17 million blind people due to cataract, and the importance of this problem being determined for ophthalmologic practice [141, 142].

The presence of such tendency is worsened by absence of effective conservative methods of prevention and treatment of age cataract and also by the high cost of the most effective at present time surgical methods of its treatment, which at the same time are not lacking of some complications. Due to these reasons, in some developing countries, only 10% patients are operated on; e.g., in Africa, there number three million blind patients with cataract, who have no financial means for surgical treatment [119].

Clinically, two main kinds of age cataract of a human being – cortical and nuclear – are distinguished. Clinical manifestations of cortical and nuclear kinds of age cataract have no great resemblance. They resemble each other only in the time of origin (at the age over 60) and the progressing decrease of visual acuity due to the gradual transparency loss of the lens. Much of the number of important clinical distinctions of cortical and nuclear kinds of age cataract is of great importance.

Modern ophthalmology also distinguishes the whole number of important peculiarities of clinical course and character of possible complications in the given kinds of age cataract (pseudoexfoliative syndrome, secondary glaucoma, fibrosis of the posterior capsule of the lens, loss of the vitreous body, instable position of the intraocular lens). The mentioned data allow supposing that the influence of such a causative factor as age on the human lens can be realized through absolutely various pathogenic mechanisms, resulting in formation of this or that kind of age cataract in the future.

The definite role of humoral system in regulation of lens epithelial cells' functioning is known. Particularly, it is shown that both excess and lack of several hormones, e.g., glucocorticoids, are accompanied by lens opacity [42, 74].

The great importance of the endocrine system in regulation of various characteristics of lenticular cells is also confirmed by the fact that these cells express the great number of receptors, e.g., H_1-histamino – [32, 146]; M_1-cholino – [45], M_3-cholino – [31]; P_2U-, P_2Y_2-purino – and α_1-adreno – receptors [30]; mineralocorticoidal receptors [126]; glucocorticoidal receptors [74]; receptors to sex hormones – estrogenic, progesteronic, androgenic [72, 73, 198]; as well as signal receptors of the epidermal growth factor [195] and many others [143, 195].

That's why the humoral system dysfunction of the body should be considered as one of the possible causes of cataract's origin, the possible role of which in regulation of various structural-and-functional characteristics of the lens, including different kinds formation of age cataract, is practically not investigated.

One more little investigated aspect of humoral regulation of the lens' functioning is its supply with biogenic amines. Investigation of their possible roles is especially actual, taking into account the described role of bioamines, e.g., histamine, in transporting regulation of calcium ions through the cellular membranes, the excess of which in lens cells is known to be able to initiate the development of one of the form of cataract [113].

Being universal hormone-mediators of nervous, endocrine and immune systems, biogenic amines take part in the great number of regulatory processes in the body [4, 41, 64, 67, 75, 79, 95, 171]; they undoubtedly participate in regulation of various structural and functional characteristics of the lens, though mechanism of such influences is not enough investigated.

In spite of great number of works dealing with the investigation of pathogenesis and treatment of cataract, morphological aspects of its origin and the possible role of bioamines state change of lens cells in the age cataract pathogenesis of a human being are not investigated.

Another aspect that is not investigated enough is that of the age cataract pathogenesis being the question of trophic function of the nervous system, being one of the most important questions in actual biological problem of stability maintenance factors of tissue differentiation and tissue metabolism of living organisms. Morphological aspects of tissue differentiation of lens cells in condition of its pathological aging in formation of various kinds of age cataract are practically not investigated.

The importance of the nervous regulatory mechanisms disturbances in pathology development is difficult to overestimate. It is known that the influence of the nervous system is exerted directly or indirectly on all the processes in the body, and nervous and psychic factors are of great importance in diseases' origin and their treatments. In his time, N.I. Pirogov already noted that wounds in soldiers of recessive army were healing slower than in soldiers-victors.

Modern literature dealing with investigation of age changes of trophic influence of the nervous system is rather extensive [135, 173, 194]; it discovers important mechanisms of many age diseases' formation. It is possibly the systemic approach to the investigation of clinic and histological state of aged people, suffering from lens opacity that allows revealing significant pathogenic mechanisms of age cataract.

Structural reactions of the eye's tissue on different influences were investigated many times [145, 178, 181, 205]. However, these works are only the tail's registration, as the reveal stable structural reorganization, supplying adaptation to the effect of damaging factors. Initial stages of adaptation in the form of temporary ("launching") functional system creation [125] were not investigated by morphologists.

The detailed qualitative and quantitative characteristics of bioamines profile of the intact human lens and lens affected by different kinds of age cataract is first presented in the given monograph.

The results of comparative immunohistochemical investigation of lens cells' phenotype in normal and in different kinds of formations of human age cataract are first mentioned.

Chapter I

Development, Structure and Regeneration of the Lens

1.1. Embryonic Development and Growth of the Lens

The development of the lens is closely connected with formation and transformation of the ocular vesicles, which are laid about three weeks after fertilization in the form of two evaginations of the cerebral part of the nervous tube on the level of the anterior cerebral vesicle [76].

Ocular vesicles grow in the direction of ectoderm, keeping connection with the nervous tubule through ocular stalks; their cavities are connected through the channel of each stalk [93]. During the ocular vesicle's growing to cerebral ectoderm, the layer comprising it in differential cubic cells begins intensively multiplying and forming multilayer thickening – the lenticular placode.

Between the lenticular placode and the ocular vesicle, the spatial connections appear, and ultramicroscopic cytoplasmic processes are formed [123]. Between the ocular vesicle and the lens embryo, there are few mesodermal cells and the intercellular fibrillary matrix giving the positive reaction on laminin and fibronectin.

On the fifth week of embryogenesis due to the invagination of distal wall, the ocular vesicle is transformed into the double-walled eyecup. Later, pigmented epithelium of the retina and the iris are developed from the external wall [112], and from the internal one – other layers of the retina. While multiplying, placoda's cells are plunged under ectoderm, forming the lens fosse, which while deepening is enclosed into the lenticular vesicle on the fifth week of embryogenesis [3, 93]. The ocular vesicle loses connection with ectoderm and is located inside the eyecup of rounded shape. Lower animals have such shape of the lens during their whole lives, and in higher animals and human beings, the lens, while being thickened, later takes the shape of the biconvex lens; in a human being, it already occurs after his birth [93].

Cell division is firstly observed through the whole ocular vesicle [77], and then mitosis is revealed only in its external, directed to the ectodermic wall, while cells of the internal wall cease premitotic synthesis of deoxyribonucleic acid (DNA) and are not divided. The wall of the ocular vesicle is presented as one layer: in the anterior part – cubic, in the posterior one – prismatic. At the end of the sixth week, cells of the posterior surface of the vesicle begin lengthening, transforming into the primary fibers. Bases of the primary fibers are adjacent to the posterior half of the capsule, and apexes reach quickly epithelial cells of anterior half of the capsule, thus by 6½ weeks, its whole cavity is filled [3, 15]. These fibers are elongated differentiated cells, the nuclei of which are gradually resorbed, mitochondria disappear, and fibers themselves, while thickening, on the ninth week form the embryo of the embryonic nucleus of the lens, which gradually becomes larger [3, 112].

The thickening of the primary fibers, according to I.F. Kovalev (1967, 1969) [98, 99], results in volume decrease of the lens substance and as a result, to tension weakening of its capsule, which is compensated for by new fibers formation, known already as secondary. Thus, in the beginning of embryonic development of the lens, the mechanism of its physiological regeneration is put into action, which is functioning during all its life. Secondary fibers formation begins on the eighth to ninth weeks and then gradually becomes slower during postnatal ontogenesis, ceasing practically only in extreme old age. The source of such fiber formation is epithelial cells of the anterior capsule. In the embryonic and early postembryonic periods of development, these cubic cells are multiplied under the whole anterior capsule, being strongly close to the equator [112]. Fiber endings grow in direction to the external and internal poles of the lens.

New layers of differentiated fibers are pushed aside the capsule by earlier formed layers, forming at the end of the second month and in the middle of the third one of embryogenesis the posterior and anterior lens sutures or stars [16].

In the embryonic period, the lens becomes fully deprived of innervations and blood vessels; however the vascular coat of the lens, performing trophic function to it, is formed from the vascularized mesenchyma around its bursa. It has blood supply through the artery of the vitreous body and is the most developed from the second to sixth month of embryogenesis and then is gradually reduced to birth. And although in many vertebrate animals the vascular coat of the lens is lacking, its existence was established in rats, rabbits and mice [3].

Further postembryonic growth of the lens is due to cells of anterior epithelium, which in the equatorial region continue differentiating into lens cells-fibers and under the capsule are added to periphery of the lens just behind the equator. Epithelial cells of the lens, proliferating and moving to the equator, serve for formation of new lens fibers. The given fact is confirmed by results of modern immunohistochemichal investigations of the lens. Intracellular distribution of the lens epithelial growth factor was investigated by means of monoclonal antibodies [32]. At the same time, immunopositivity is maximal in the nuclei of central lens epithelial cells, being less marked in the nuclei of equatorial epithelial ones.

The same growth factor in less concentration also presents in cytoplasm of lens epithelial cells and superficial cells-fibers. The author tends to connect concentration decrease of the epithelial growth factor of the lens in its nucleus with terminal differentiation process, which has certain resemblance with biochemical mechanisms of apoptosis [32].

Lens fibers as well as epithelial cells participating in its formation are kept during the whole life. The lens doesn't lose fibers, consequently cellular change doesn't take place.

Before becoming a fiber, an epithelial cell has the nucleus and the greater part of common cytoplasmatic organelles. In the cell-fiber transformation into lens fiber, its nuclear chromatin and nucleoli disappear, the nuclear coat forms vesicles and then is very likely to be dissolved. From all cytoplasmatic organelles, only clusters of free ribosomes and several longitudinally located microtubules are kept. On electronic microphoto, the rest fibers look granular and have characteristic for lens fibers' proteins – crystallines [76].

1.2. Morphogenic Influences and Induction of the Lens

"Directed differentiation of ectodermic presumptive epithelium in the lens is the result of successive morphogenic influences exerted by the ocular vesicle, the eyecup and later by the retina, the exerted influence of which is called as initiating since the time of H. Speman (1901, 1905) and W.H. Lewis (1904)" (quotation according to E.V. Maltsev and K.P. Pavluchenko, 2002) [119].

It must be noted that under the inducing influence of neuroectodermic embryo of the eye (ocular vesicle), the ectodermic lenticular placode also acquires properties of neuroectodermic tissue and is not common epithelium [193]. That's why epithelial cells of the lens under certain pathological conditions (e.g., subcapsular cataracts) are able to form the fibrous tissue, containing collagenous fibers [119].

By experiments on animals and birds, it is shown that primary fibers are differentiated only from these epithelial cells of the lenticular vesicle, which are directed to the retina's embryo; and the existence of special mechanism controlling the size, form and orientation of the developing lens is proved. On hens' embryo of five days, these investigators established that if to carry on an inversion of the lens, i.e., surgically turn it by anterior epithelium to the neural retina, the lengthening of those cells of the posterior wall, which had already begun differentiating, ceased. However, from epithelium, directed now to the retina embryo, new primary fibers are differentiated [119].

Nowadays, it is supposed that induction is performed by means of chemical factors, produced by an inductor of the lens, under the influence of which the lens is laid, and then cells' transition of its epithelium to the equatorial zone, their lengthening, dislocation into the cortex and also further differentiating of fibers, accompanied by the nuclei loss, take place.

"D. Barritault et al. (1980) separated from the bull's retina the albuminous growth factor with molecular weight of about 5,000. By its addition in concentration of 1mcg/ml into cultural fluid proliferation of not only epithelial cells of the lens, but a number of others (endothelium of vessels, myoblasts, chondrocytes, keratinocytes), except fibroblasts, is stimulated. The same authors reported that cells morphology of the bull's lens in culture was changed from purely epithelial into fibroblast-like under the influence of that factor. In such cells, many microtubules are formed, and between neighboring ones – interrupted junctions are formed. Cells continue actively synthesizing sulphated glycosaminoglycans, connected with the lens capsule formation" (quotation according to E.V. Maltsev et al., 2002) [119].

One of the mentioned factors, formed by neuroretina, is the growth factor of fibroblasts [116]. The growth factor of fibroblasts has high concentration in the vitreous body and low – in chamber humor [115, 124]. In epithelium explanation of the lens central zone of newborn rats in nutrient medium, containing the mentioned factor of retina, multilayer formations from elongated cells are formed and synthesis of β- and γ-crystallines takes place [147]. Under the influence of the same factor, the cells of the central zone of anterior epithelium lose with age the ability of differentiating into fibers [148].

Except the growth factor of fibroblasts, the lens fibers differentiating is controlled by other growth factors, separated by retina: the epidermal growth factor and the insulin-like growth factor. The mentioned growth factors have peptide nature. In cultivation of epithelial cells of the human lens in nutrient medium, they act in very low concentrations – about 10^{-2}-10^2 ng/ml [83, 84].

It is experimentally proved [119] that in the early stages of embryogenesis practically any of its sites has ability to induce influence perception of the ocular vesicle, except lens-forming ectoderm. That's why the ocular vesicle implantation under ectoderm of other sites of the developing embryo's body or ectodermic sites transplantation into the ocular vesicles region result in normal lens' development. However, while the embryo is developing, the potential ability of ectoderm to transform into the lens keeps only in lens-forming ectoderm.

1.3. Lens' Regeneration in Vertebrate Animals and a Human Being

The lens possesses certain ability to regenerate, to repeated (secondary) development, caused by its injury. Full-value of reparation in different kinds of animals is greatly varied – from reparation of not large defects to complete lens restoration instead of lost one.

Biologists established long ago that among vertebrate animals, Amphibia caudate has maximal ability to regeneration. For example, according to G. Wolff (1895), in triton the complete regeneration of the full-value lens instead of the lost one occurs. The process of its secondary development is termed "Wolff's regeneration" of the lens, named after one of the pioneers investigating this phenomenon.

A characteristic feature of Wolff's regeneration lies in that the lens regenerates from the ocular iris, which being a derivative of the nervous tube, while in embryogenesis, the source for the lens development is skin ectoderm. Hence, in the given case, cellular metaplasia of one kind into another takes place. The process of Wolff's regeneration completes in a month by development of the full-value lens and has 13 stages, grouped into four periods [119].

In several Amphibia ecaudata and amblistom (Rana esculenta, Rana dalmatina, Discoglossus pictus), the new lens is restored from a fragment of the old one [12].

In tadpoles of Xenopus laevis, the source of lens regeneration is corneal epithelium, forming rounded cells, transforming into new lens by ontogenetic-like way [13]. Regeneration frequency at the same time reaches 90% [14]. In larvae of Xenopus laevis, the sclera is also able to regenerate lens, controlled by retina [14].

The stimulating influence of biogenic amine (histamine) on mitotic activity of lens epithelial cells of a rat was described; the attempt to disclose mechanisms of bioamines regulation of regeneration process of the lens after chemical irritation of an eye was made [96, 97].

Unfortunately, in a human being and mammal animals, full-value lens regeneration doesn't occur either after its different injuries (pathological morphology of cataracts) or after its removal (secondary cataract). It is secondary cataract that in 22.5% cases complicates extracapsular extraction of the lens, being an example of atypical regeneration, resulting in incomplete restoration of the organ [107].

Clinically, we mark out the following varieties of secondary cataract: 1 – the posterior wall thickening of the capsule; 2 – Elscnig's balls formation on the posterior capsule surface; 3 – diffusive and local fibrosis of the lens posterior capsule [18].

By means of light, transmission and scanning electronic microscopy, it was confirmed that the single source of Elscnig's balls formation is lens epithelial cells [199].

Several epithelial cells acquire elongated and dendritic shape and also the ability to proliferate and migrate [49, 106]. The same cells possess ability to produce the intracellular matrix, containing collagen [81, 130], presented by its I, IV, V and VI types [129]. It is disclosed that metaplastic cells of lens epithelium acquired ability to contractility [82], which is supplied by synthesis of α-smooth muscular actin in these lens cells [103, 155].

Epithelial cells contractility is able to produce capsule contraction, resulting in formation of some postoperative complications, initiating retinal detachment and decentration of the intraocular lens [103, 104, 155]. That's why some authors are inclined to call metaplastic cells myofibroblasts [80, 82].

It is proved that both myofibroblastic transformation of lens epithelial cells in secondary cataract development and loss of some of them by apoptosis are controlled by one and the same growth factor – the transforming growth factor β (TGF$_β$) [92]. The given property of the mentioned growth factor may be used with the purpose of secondary cataract prophylaxis by means of apoptosis induction of lens epithelial cells. According to the latest data [202], in epithelium of the human lens, obtained in capsulorexis during age cataract extraction, apoptosis frequency reaches 1.7%.

The lens with its apparent simplicity of structure is the rather complex biological structure and is worthy of rapt detailed investigation on the basis of the fact that it keeps transparency in most people. even of declining years. The possibility of spontaneous resorption of traumatic floriform cataract is described. In some cases (98 similar cases were described), the phenomenon of complete spontaneous resorption of lens masses with capsular integrity keeping and visual functions restoration is developed [11, 137-139].

Chapter II

The Human Lens Normally and in Age Cataract Formation

2.1. Macro-and Microscopic Structure of the Intact Human Lens

The lens of an adult human being is transparent, slightly yellowish, semisolid body in the form of biconvex lens with diameter from 9 to 10 mm and thickness from 3.6 to 5 mm depending on accommodation. The lens is isolated from other ocular membranes by the capsule, doesn't contain nerves or vessels [50], thus explaining impossibility of inflammatory processes in the lens. According to the power of refraction, the lens is the second medium (after cornea) of optic system of the eye. Its refracting power averages 19.11 dptr, in maximal accommodation tension – 33.06 dptr [177]. In newborns, the lens is of ball-shaped form and has mild consistence and refracting power up to 35.0 dptr. In the eye, the lens is located between the iris and the vitreous body, in the deepening on the anterior surface of the latter. It is kept in this position by fibers of the supporting ligament (zonula ciliaris), which by their other ending are attached to the inner surface of the ciliary body.

Lens consistency is mild in young years. Density of its central part is increased with age. In the lens, one distinguishes the equator and two poles – anterior and posterior. Along the equator, the lens is conditionally divided into the anterior and posterior surfaces. The line, connecting the anterior and posterior poles, is called the lens axis. The anterior surface of the lens is less convex than the posterior one. The anterior and posterior surfaces of the lens are washed by aqueous humor.

Histologically in the lens, one distinguishes the capsule (capsule of lens) and its substance (substance of lens), consisting of the lens nucleus (nucleus of lens) and its cortex (cortex of lens).

The inner surface of the lens anterior capsule is lined with monolayer epithelium, performing trophic, barrier and cambial functions [177].

Cells of anterior epithelium of the lens have hexagonal form; at the equator they acquire elongated form and are transformed into lens fibers (fibers of lens).

"Fibers formation takes place during the whole life of a human being, resulting in volume increase of the lens. However, over increase doesn't take place, as central older fibers lose water, become dense and gradually form compact nucleus in the centre" (quotation according to Eroshevsky T.I. et al., 1977) [50].

This phenomenon of age sclerosing of the lens, which is clinically evident by the distance of the closest point of clear vision, should be considered a physiological process, resulting in only volume decrease of accommodation, but practically doesn't decrease lenticular transparency.

It has been recently noticed that depolarization processes, resulting in structural organization disturbance of the lens, take place with age, and that, in its turn, changes radius of its curvature and leads to clinical refraction change, typical for presbyopy [17].

The lens capsule is a typical basal membrane. It is structureless and strongly reflects light and is stable to different pathological factors effects. In incisions, the capsule tends to become twisted to the outside [177]. The capsule is rich in reticular fibers, except collagen and glycoproteids, usually in basal membrane, it contains sulphated glycosaminoglycan [24, 76]. When epithelial cells form the lens capsule, their plasmatic membranes are closely intertwined, and on its free surface – become dense. Here, thin plates of the fibrillar substance are gradually added to the forming capsule.

The lens is attached to the ciliary body by means of the ciliary zonule. The ciliary zonule is attached to the ciliary body on its whole length, directing to the lens equator the ciliary zonule fibers, are crossed and entwined into the lens capsule in 2 mm to front and 1 mm to behind the equator, forming the interzonular Hannover's channell [177].

2.2. Modern Data about Organization and Functioning of Lens Cells

Nowadays, investigators have a renewed interest; there appeared new technical facilities, allowing investigating biochemical, morphological and physiological processes of the eye normally and in different pathologies on a sufficiently new and higher level.

Knowledge of early stages of pathological process formation is of great importance, as on these stages there are situations that determine the character of further way of this process development and allow carrying on the necessary correction taking into account stored knowledge.

Lately, many investigations are concerned with studying the question of receptors supply of lens cells. The presence of the following receptors in cells of the intact human lens is proved: H_1-histamino – [32, 146]; M_1-cholino – [45], M_3-cholino – [31]; P_2U-, P_2Y_2-purino – and α_1-adreno – receptors [30]; mineralocorticoidal receptors [126]; glucocorticoidal receptors [74]; receptors to sex hormones–estrogenic, progesteronic, androgenic [72, 73, 198]; as well as signal receptors of the epidermal growth factor [195] and many others [143, 195].

Regional distinctions in distribution and spatial heterogeneity of functional activity of revealed receptors are described [32].

For example: M_1-cholino-receptors are located only in central cells of anterior epithelium of a lens [21, 32]; H_1-histamino-receptors are both in the central and equatorial parts of anterior epithelium of the lens.

Receptors to the epithelial growth factor (EGF) and the transforming growth factor-α (α-TGF) are revealed only in cells of the equatorial part of anterior epithelium of the lens. P_2U-, P_2Y_2-purino-receptors are both in the central part of anterior epithelium (activity is poorly marked) and in its equatorial part [32].

The given fact may serve as a case history of different degrees of functional activity of epithelial cells, located in the mentioned parts of the lens.

It is known that in women during the postmenopausal period, the risk of cataract development and retina diseases (central involutional chorioretinopathy) is greatly increased. It is experimentally proved that 17_α- and 17_β-estradiol has ability to keep normal level of adenosine triphosphoric acid (ATP), function of mitochondria and vital capacity of lens cells, even in condition of oxygen injuries of the lens [196]. Revealing of α-estrogenic receptors in different layers of the retina [133] is the important link in pathogenesis identification of the given pathology.

Various subtypes of estrogenic receptors are revealed; their subcellular distribution is described in detail. For example, α- and β-subtypes in a human being are revealed in nuclei of lens epithelial cells, as that in mitochondria of the same cells, there are only β-subtype of estrogenic receptors [19], being the evidence of their various cytoprotective potential possibility.

By means of immunofluorescence, subcellular localization of various isoforms of β-subtype of estrogenic receptors is described in detail. For example, $β_1$-subtype of estrogenic receptors is chiefly localized in mitochondria of epithelial cells of the lens; $β_2$- and $β_5$-subtypes are mainly revealed in their nuclei and cytosol [20].

M-cholino-receptors have great importance for eye's functions. Muscarinic agonists lead to the mydriatic pupil, intraocular pressure decrease, and drainage increase of aqueous humor due to muscular contraction of the ciliary body.

The ability of atropine to reduce sclera extracellular proteins production as well as the stimulating influence of carbahol on liquid part production of a tear was described. It is interesting that cholinomimetic agents in small doses activate receptors to the epidermal growth factor. Exact mechanisms of signalization are not discovered; however it is known that cholino-receptors activation is accompanied by response of lens epithelial cells as cytosolic calcium ions mobilization. This response is not of neuronal character [45].

The link between chemical irritation of ocular mucus and activation of cerebral neurons is of great interest in the view of neuro-immuno-endocrinological interactions.

In thiopental-anesthetized rats, the irritating action of some chemical substances by their application on the eyeball's surface is investigated. It is revealed that neurons' activation as a result of experimentally described effect takes place in caudal trigeminal subnucleus and depends on the dose of chemical substance. The sufficient weakening of neurons response on the contact of ocular mucus with histamine after H_1-antagonist is also shown [22].

Calcium channels are of great importance for normal metabolism supplying of the lens, as level increase of cytoplasmatic calcium in epithelial lens cells leads to functional activity stimulation and these cells' growth intensity [45]. In cortical cataract, isolated concentration increase of calcium ions takes place without simultaneous concentration change of sodium ions (in the lens, there are highly sensitive calcium channels, much more sensitive than for sodium ions).

Cells of the intact lens have very low calcium permeability, at that time calcium channels in epithelial cells have more marked activity than the same channels in fibers of lens [29]. It is noted that during cellular differentiation, lens cells lose high activity of calcium channels.

It is revealed that even minor excess of normal calcium level in epithelial lens cells initiates content increase of calcium-mobilizing antagonists in them, which support calcium channels work.

Activity of these cells is blocked by concentration decrease of outer calcium, level increase of outer potassium, several trace elements – zinc, nickel, magnesium. It is important to note that the mentioned channels of the lens appear to be inert to nifedipine's action (calcium channel blocker). Epithelial lens cells also contain tapsigargine – a substance causing stable and prolonged concentration decrease of calcium ions.

According to Williams, M.R. et al. (2001) [200], agonists and antagonists of calcium entry are kept inside the lens cell. Their system supplies signal mechanism for calcium overload prevention of the lens.

Histamine, ATP, carbachol and sulfur are referred to calcium-mobilizing agents of the lens [134].

Acetylcholine doesn't change calcium ions concentration in epithelial lens cells. Diethylstilbestrol increases calcium ions concentration in epithelial lens cells [157].

Tapsigargine induces prolonged cytoplasmatic calcium level. Other calcium-mobilizing agents influence after tapsigargine is not effective [46].

One more important factor of the lens is glutathione. It is proved that it modulates calcium channel's state indirectly through histamine release inhibition [156].

The importance of investigations in the given field is stressed by data about lens incubation into calcium-saturated medium with the purpose of modeling of one of cataract's kinds [113].

It is proved that the lens capsule possesses mechanisms of calcium signal protection system; however, M_1-cholinactivity of the lens capsule is lost after performed operation on account of cataract. Authors made a supposition about mechanism of common postoperative complication forming–econdary cataract or lens posterior capsule opacity [33].

The fact of direct dependence of metabolism character inside cell on its biomembrane's state is of common knowledge. Lipid characteristics studying of human lens fibers membranes showed high concentrations presence of cholesterol, sphingolipids [152].

Radiographic investigation of lipids organization in lens fibers membranes showed cholesterol regions location in them with definite periodicity, being equal 34Å, which corresponds to periodicity of one cell. Cholesterol regions play an important part in lens transparency supporting, as make interferences to cataractogenic aggregation of lens proteins on membrane [140].

It is proved that oxygen tension level in the lens is an important participant in age cataract development. Electronic microscopy data about lens fibers after hyperbaric oxygenation performing (HBO) shows this fact, revealing fine but important morphological structural changes of cytoplasm by the model of its reorganization in mild oxygenation, which is typical for age nuclear cataract. Hence, lens injury with HBO using may serve as the value model of age nuclear cataract [56].

In comparison with other tissues, the lens has exclusively low level of respiration. The intact lens uses and excretes the same amount of oxygen – its respiratory coefficient equals in normal 1.0 [136]. Excess of normal oxygen tension level in the lens has injurious action.

Morphological substrate, regulating oxygen influence on lens cells, was discovered in 2003, by the group of American scientists who isolated from the lens an oxygen-regulating protein (ORP 150) [69].

Glutathione is considered an important lens antioxidant [44], the level of which is sufficiently decreased in lenses, changed due to cataract.

The work by A.N. Andreev (1992) [7] is considered interesting and giving a new trend in ophthalmology, as cause-effect relations of age cataract with biogeochemical factors are disclosed in it. Dependence of age cataract development mechanism on trace elements content of environmental objects – soil, water, food – is shown. The author proved the link between cataractogenesis and increased concentrations of silicon, which are potentiated by ions of calcium, magnesium and fluorine, resulting in lipid peroxidation stimulation.

2.3. Pathological Morphology of Cataracts

Any unfavorable influence on the lens, exceeding its compensatory possibilities, initiates opacity–transparency disturbance, morphological substrate of which is combination of its various structural dystrophic and necrotic changes. Pathomorpological picture of the lens in sufficiently developed opacity, including the old one, contains changes of fibers, epithetlium and capsule.

Fibers of the lens with opacity are swollen, homogenized and disintegrated with formation of amorphous and small-grained detritus, larger rounded eosinophilic Morgagnian balls, which arise in the swelling of fibers fragments and then are diluted [170].

Young fibers, locating on the equator and in the posterior cortical layer under the capsule, due to wrong differentiation acquire form of vacuolated pear-shaped Vedl's cells, the nuclei of which have common sizes [188]. Correct location of the nuclei on equator of lens along the nuclear arch is disturbed, and then the nuclear arch is not determined at all, as Vedl's cells are chaotically located instead of it. Crystals of cholesterol and lime can be located in the lens detritus [51, 144].

As early as 1907, C. Hess paid attention to lens epithelium changes in cataractogenesis. Located side by side, cells have different sizes; their nuclei are picnotized, enlarged, polymorphous and disintegrated into separate fragments, cytoplasm of epithelial cells are vacuolized [10].

In the process of lens opacity formation, against presenting diabetes mellitus of II type in particular, location density decrease of epithelial cells in the preequatorial zone from 4370 in normal to 3745 per mm^2 is noted [180].

The fact of fibrous structures formation with tinctorial properties of collagen by epithelial lens cells is of special interest; at the same time superficial resemblance of mentioned cells with fibroblasts is noted [10, 101, 102]. According to D. Kurosaka et al. (1996) [104], S. Saika et al. (1997) [155] and others, such metaplased cells possess ability to produce a marker of myofibroblasts – α-smooth muscular actin.

In rare cases due to lyze of diluted cortical masses of the lens and its nucleus, the visual function restoration can take place. This phenomenon is called as spontaneous resorption of age cortical cataract in the course of its hypermaturing (Morgagnian cataract).

Sometimes in age cataract hypermaturing, vice versa, excessive thickening of the whole lens substance is observed, detritus is located between sclerosed fibers; hard, black cataract is formed [10]. Predominance of fibers thickening over their disintegration distinguishes black nuclear age cataract from gray cortical one.

Pathological changes of the lens capsule in the course of cataractogenesis are concluded in formation of, except true exfoliation, also pseudoexfoliation, first described by Lindberg in 1917. This term means the state in which the capsule isn't degraded and on its anterior surface, the papillary margin and posterior surface of the iris, the cilliary processes and zonular fibers there appear deposits, containing glycogen, mucopolysaccharides and tyrosine.

The result of pseudoexfoliation of lens capsule is glaucoma, associated with age (commonly of nuclear type) cataract [23, 91].

N.I. Kurysheva (2001) distinguishes four times much more frequent loss of the vitreous body and instable location of the intraocular lens in patients with age nuclear cataract pseudoexfoliative superpositions [100].

"Nowadays many investigators confirm the point of view concerning pseudoexfoliative syndrome as on systemic disturbance, being the result of multifocal metabolic process of unknown pathology, resulting in primary changes of cells and characterized by fibrilliary material accumulation, which contain components of basal membranes" (quotation according to E.V. Maltsev and K.P. Pavluchenko, 2002) [119].

Protein fibrillin in large number is contained in pseudoexfoliative material fibers, where was discovered by homogeneous antibodies U. Schlotzer-Schrehardt et al. (1997), locating directly among cellular organelles [159].

Scanning and transmission electronic microscopy shows the following cataractogenic changes sequence: the number decrease of normal contact between cells-fibers of the lens, their wrinkling, lacuna forming, lens fibers edema and fissure formation, membrane destruction, fibrillary orientation disturbance and their replacement by amorphous material [189].

2.4. Modern Point of View on Age Cataract Pathogenesis

Considerable morphological and clinical distinctions of main varieties of age cataract (cortical and nuclear), especially on early stages of forming, are of common knowledge, clinical and morphological manifestations of which have no great resemblance [119].

For the cortical kind of age cataract, it is characteristic to have aqueous fissure appearing, dissociation of cortex, accumulating in extracellular space by humor (according to V. Happe (2005), "extracellular cataract") [78]. Further, there takes place opacity of aqueous fissure and forming of larger pin-like opacity, which gradually moves in direction of anterior and posterior lens capsules, and on the stage of mature cortical cataract, the whole cortex is subjected to opacity, acquiring white color ("gray" cataract).

In nuclear kind, formation of age cataract primary opacity appears in the internal embryonic nucleus of the lens and cytoplasm of the lens cells (according to V. Happe (2005), "intracellular cataract") [78], distributing then on all parts of mature nucleus. Opacity has reddish or reddish black color ("brown" cataract), has homogenous character and is diffusely located [141].

Nowadays, the process of lens opacity is considered as a multifactorial and polyethiological disease. At the same time, it is important to note that about 85% cases of cataract disease are caused by age cataract [119], pathogenic mechanisms of which is impossible to consider exact today. Interaction between age cataract morbidity increase and increased fluorine concentrations in drinking water [119] and also from the whole complex of biogeochemical factors [182] was established.

The presence of certain common diseases of the body (essential hypertension, diseases of liver, gastrointestinal tract, hyperglycemia and others) also increases the risk of age cataract development in a concrete patient [184].

Investigators of different countries pay great attention to radiation factors, initiating cataractogenesis (sunlight's effect). As it is known [110], solar radiation, reaching Earth's surface, has spectrum from 250 up to 1800 nm. In its content, there is 2% ultraviolet radiation, 40% visible radiation and 58% infrared radiation. Radiation causes photoinjury of those ocular tissues only that absorb it. Light in the range of wave length from 480 to 1200nm is not practically absorbed by ocular optical medium, and, hence, probability of optical medium photoinjury is small. However, it sharply increases in radiation effect with wave length shorter than 480 nm, i.e., in blue and ultraviolet parts of spectrum. This part of spectrum is especially dangerous for retina photoreceptors. Light shorter than 300-310 nm is absorbed by the cornea, and the lens of old people practically doesn't transmit ultraviolet part of spectrum. After surgical removal of cataract, a barrier from ultraviolet rays is eliminated, and prerequisites for retina photoinjury are created.

R.A. Weale (1987) pointed at more frequent origin of age cataract in people of south regions of the globe [197].

Ultraviolet light with wave length of 280-315 nm, i.e., irradiation of B range, is especially dangerous for the lens. At the same time, it is characteristic that people being subjected to such irradiation for a long-term period fall ill with cataract of the cortical type more frequently [36, 37], regardless of sex and race.

Cortical opacity appears more frequently in infranasal quadrant of the lens (57%), prevailing over opacity in three others its quadrants, taken together [158], which shows penetration of the most part of light energy into the eye directly from atmosphere, the least part is reflected from surface of water, snow or sand.

E.V. Larionov et al. (1989) [106] experimentally proved the possibility of posterior lens capsule injuries by immune complexes of lens antigens – antibodies, which cause cells appearing with fibroblasts morphology and fibrosis. Posterior capsule injury by immunoglobulins is possible even on paired eye [54]. It is known that posterior capsule integrity disturbance causes more serious disturbances of ionic homeostasis of the lens than injury of the anterior one [55].

It is established that in cataract in patients with myopia, the anterior lens capsule becomes thin, and the posterior one, vice versa, is subjected to more thickening than in emmetrops [47].

In patients with myopia, tendency of the lens capsule to collagen fibers aggregation is also described [150, 151].

Investigation of ultrastructural disturbances of the lens with scanning electronic microscopy applying in conditions of nuclear cataract development in old patients revealed in the lens the regions formation of its "globular degeneration." They consist of spherical protein globules (multilamellar bodies, MLBs) with diameter from 1 to 20 mcm, covered by two-layer lipid membrane, and they are able to decrease optical transmission to 65% [61, 62]. Besides, granules of glycogen with size of 25-35 nm are revealed [121]. Described pathological changes received numerous confirmations in investigations carried on by other authors' collectives [34, 57].

It is proved that human MrgX3 gene, transplanted into transgenic rats, causes normal process interruption of cellular differentiation and results in cataract formation, accompanied by watering of the lens, swelling and degeneration of its cells-fibers [88].

The state of sex hormones and their receptors in patients with age cataract was studied in detail.

An attempt to find out the mechanism of high cataract morbidity in women in postmenopausal period resulted in discovering of estrogenic protection of mitochondrial function of epithelial lens cells and ATP level in oxidizing injury process, which increases vital capacity of lens cells by 95% [196].

At that time, it is noted that estrogen has great importance in physiology of the lens of both sexes [38]. According to other investigators [108, 204], sex hormone levels may be considered as risk factors only for cataract formation but not as the key factor.

Among a number of mentioned literature sources, the great interest has been in an article of group of Japan investigators-ophthalmologists. It confirms that under the influence of injuring factors, epithelial lens cells enter the process of epithelial-and-mesenchymal transition and under control of the transforming growth factor β_2 (TGF-β_2) are subjected to transformation into myofibroblasts, positive for established marker of this process [153, 154].

Data, obtained by this authors' collective, are conformed and logically add to the results obtained by scientific associates of other laboratories in different times during independent scientific investigations. For example, "special interest in several cataracts has the fact of forming of fibrous structures with tinctorial properties of collagen at outer resemblance of these cells with fibroblasts by epithelial lens cells. This phenomenon was first described already in 1906 by R. Onfray, Opin..." (quotation according to E.V. Maltsev et al., 2002) [119]. The similar phenomenon is described in cataract, combining with primary glaucoma [101, 102]. An experimental model of cataract formation, based on TGF-β_2 (transforming growth factor β_2) influence, inducing appearance of epithelial-and-mesenchymal transition in lens cells, was suggested [39].

Metaplasia of epithelial lens cells remained after extracapsular extraction of cataract (ECEC), and forming by them collagen result in lens capsule fibrosis – varieties of secondary cataract [129-131]. Furthermore, according to Kurosaka D. et al. (1996) [104] and Saika S. et al. (1997) [155], such metaplased cells are able to produce a marker of myofibroblasts – α-actin of smooth muscular cells (α-SMA) as well as to manifest in some cases positivity for pancytokeratin and vimentin or for vimentin only [183].

Due to the described properties, lens cells can produce lens capsule contraction, which promotes the forming of some intra- and postoperative complications – lens posterior capsule rupture, vitreous body prolapse, retinal detachment, intraocular lens decentration [104, 155] and others.

For this reason, a number of authors tend to call metaplased cells myofibroblasts [80, 82] or mesenchymal cells [183]. As a result of these cells plasticity, allowing performing the process of epithelial-and-mesenchymal transition, and regardless of phenotype, cells acquire various functional defects [128].

In 2003, in the journal *Curr Opin Cell Biology*, there was published a review by J.P. Thiery (Curie's Institute, France) [185], in which prevalence, mechanisms and physiological essence of the given process were described in detail.

Epithelial-and-mesenchymal transition (EMT) is recognized as fundamental process, regulating morphogenesis in multicellular organisms. This process is reactivated in different diseases, including fibrosis [160] and malignant neoplasm progressing [128].

Molecular mechanisms EMT, primarily studied on epithelial cells culture, resulted in "transduction trunks" discovering [185], leading to epithelial cells polarity loss and acquiring a number of mesenchymal phenotypic signs (epithelial markers decrease).

Analogous mechanisms are repeatedly described in vivo in the course of physiological development of multicellular organisms, e.g., in the period of gastrulation [174].

According to data of A.Y. Demir et. al. (2004) [40], menstruation influences on mesothelial cells' morphology, launching in them energo-dependent transition process of epithelial phenotype into mesenchymal one. For example, expression decrease of cytokeratin, fibrillar actin, α-tubulin, constantly high expression of vimentin and expression decrease of E-cadherin are described. Besides, intracellular contacts changes and motility increase of mesothelial cells are revealed. All the described changes have reversible character.

Epithelial-and-mesenchymal transdifferentiating was also described in renal fibrosis, arising against a background of glomerulonephritis [9]. Authors carried on detailed studying of phenotypical characteristics of cellular changes, typical to renal fibrosis, on the basis of which the following conclusion was made: "epithelial-and-mesenchymal transdifferentiating – is the transient cellular phenomenon, presented also in human renal globule, promoting myofibroblasts formation from epithelial cells and fibrosis development in renal globules" (quotation according to Bariety J. et al., 2003) [9].

On culture of lens epithelial cells, it was proved [153] that shortly after injury, the signal transformer (Smad3) of the transforming growth factor-β was activated. Authors show that blocking of the mentioned transductor results in decrease of phenotypical changes of lens epithelial cells in the course of "epithelial-and-mesenchymal transition (EMT)," blocking markers expression of EMT (α-smooth muscular actin, collagen of I type). Authors raised a supposition that "blocking of Smad3-trunk can be useful for fibrosis inhibition of the lens capsule after surgical injury."

Chapter III

Biogenic Amines Role in the Functioning of Eye's Tissues

Nowadays, biogenic amines influence on functioning of many tissues of human and animal organisms is investigated in detail [41, 94, 95, 117, 175, 173, 85-87].

Their active participation as neurotransmitters of the central nervous system was proved [43, 48, 65, 66, 68, 71, 161-169, 191, 192, 201], in circadian rhythms system [1, 2].

The humoral system role in regulation of various structural and functional characteristics of lens tissues is practically not investigated. The importance of bioamines influence on functioning processes of lens cells is confirmed by the presence of large number of receptors to bioamines.

3.1. Histamine Influence on Eye's Tissues

Many tissues of the human and animal eye – the iris, the ciliary body, the lens, the vascular membrane, the retina, the sclera and the optic nerve – were tested on account of histamine quantitative content [96, 132]. For all that, maximal concentrations of the given diamine were revealed in the vascular membrane, minimal – in the retina.

Authors registered histamine level increase in ocular tissues in certain kinds of its pathology – endophthalmitis, glaucoma, penetrating wound of the eye and so on.

In the lens of the human eye, a type of predominating histamine receptor was determined. It is shown that calcium ions mobilization in cytoplasm of lens epithelial cells, caused by histamine, is blocked by triprolidin (H_1-blocker) but isn't changed under the influence of H_2- and H_3-antagonists [32, 127, 146]. The given fact allows confirming that lens cells on their surface chiefly have H_1- receptors.

Studying of local distinctions in functional receptors localization to bioamines (histamine, acetylcholine) in the intact human lens showed the presence of important functional distinctions between central and equatorial epithelial cells of the lens [32].

Functional activity level was estimated according to concentration change of the epithelial growth factor (EGF). Authors testify to considerable concentration increase of the given growth factor in response to histamine injection both in central and equatorial epithelial cells of the lens. Acetylcholine injection is accompanied by considerable EGF level increase in central epithelial cells, while equatorial epithelial cells remain indifferent. The above-described reactions are canceled by blockers of H_1-, M_1-, $P_2Y_{(2)}$-receptors, that is the evidence of the presence of the mentioned receptors on lens cells surface [32].

The given data show the modeling influence of biogenic amines, including histamine, on the growth indices of lens cells. Their growth intensity is connected with mobilization degree of cytoplasmatic calcium, which is stimulated by injected histamine [46]. Hence, histamine is one of calcium-mobilizing agents [134].

The group of investigators under supervision of Lui P.P. in 2003, published an article with detailed description of physiological influence of histamine on cellular division. By means of confocal and electronic microscopy, arising dynamic changes of mitochondria and nuclear tubules (double membranes, nuclear membrane invagination, connected with nucleus) in response to histamine stimulation were revealed, which were consequently included into specialized dynamic regulation process of calcium in cellular nuclei [118].

Histamine level in the lens is very variable and depends on many factors. For example, minor exceeding of normal concentration of calcium ions in lens epithelial cells results in increase of histamine level in them – activation of calcium-mobilizing agents takes place [200].

High concentration of calcium ions results in synthesis de novo of highly molecular polymers and molecules of β-crystalline (M=55000), which don't occur in normal lens [58].

For all that, it is shown that formation of the mentioned pathological protein (β-crystalline) is blocked by histamine [114].

Thus modern data, characterizing histamine role in exchange processes of the lens, is the evidence of both its participation in the course of pathological process and importance of histamine properties, directed to participation processes of cellular division and also to fight with cataractogenesis.

3.2. Catecholamine Influence on Eye's Tissues

In the studied literature, there is scanty information about various α-adrenergic substances influence on tissues of the human eyeball [63, 120].

It is proved that not all mydriatic means applied in ophthalmology have the same physiological effects.

For example, dophaminergic mean (2% ibopamin) possesses more marked mydriatic effect than α-adrenomimetic (10% phenylephrine) and M-cholino-blocker (1% tropicamide). However, applying of just α-adrenomimetic (10% phenylephrine) doesn't result in intraocular pressure increase even in patients suffering from glaucoma simplex [120].

It is known that applying of dophaminergic mean (2% ibopamin) is accompanied by intraocular pressure level increase only in eyes with glaucoma simplex [63]; that's why it is suggested to use the revealed effect for the purpose of practical ophthalmology as provocation test in glaucoma simplex diagnostics. Mechanism of the revealed effects isn't described at present.

From the point of view of age cataract pathogenesis, data about mechanisms of various complicated cataracts formation are of interest. For example, cortical cataract, manifested by swelling, exfoliation and disintegration of fibers, arises after protamine and adrenaline injection into rabbit's body and also in experimental hemorrhage in the vitreous body.

According to L.E. Cherikchi (1990, 1992), L.E. Cherikchi et al. (1993, 1994) [25-28], pathological chemical correlations between the vitreous body and the lens determine preliminary accumulation of products of protein disintegration, sugar, histamine and other substances in the vitreous body, leading then to their redistribution and accumulation in lens posterior layers.

In the lens capsule and in the region of its anterior epithelium, the presence of β-adreno-receptors is revealed [5, 6]. It is proved that the mentioned receptors stimulation is accompanied by lens capsule permeability increase.

It is revealed that oxytocin exerts the marked stimulating influence on noradrenergic receptors of various tissues. For all that, oxytocin production is considerably increased by norepinephrin and histamine [111].

The revealed data are evidence of importance and variety of manifestations connected with physiological effects realization of catecholamine in ocular tissue.

3.3. Serotonin Influence on Eye's Tissues

Serotonin biogenic amines influence on eyeball's tissue is investigated in more detail.

In vivo et in vitro, circadian rhythms of serotonin level in the lens of experimental animals with the maximum of concentrations in the wakeful state period are described.

It is established that N-acetyltransferase serotonin is the key ferment in melatonin biosynthesis, revealed in the laboratory rat's lens [2]. It points at the existence of more important biosynthesis mechanisms in animals, not depending on light conditions in periods of sleep and wakeful state.

It is proved that N-acetylserotonin is an indirect precursor of melatonin, able to catch free radicals and prevent macromolecules (proteins, fats, nuclear and mitochondrial DNA) from oxidative injury in all subcellular structures. Consequently, practical application of N-acetylserotonin with the purpose of maximal realization of melatonin antioxidant properties must be accompanied by detailed investigation of their physiological effects [203].

It must be noted that melatonin is an important marker of just age pathology [105].

Melatonin, besides hormonal effects, as other biogenic amines, possesses neurotransmitteral functions. Possibility of extrapineal synthesis of melatonin by endocrine and nonendocrine cells of different localizations, including some endothelial cells, is considered to be proved at present [105].

It is proved that serotonin changes the course of amacrine retinal cells development, increases intraocular pressure level, causes ocular blood vessels constriction, and causes papillary constriction [60].

Serotonin physiological influences on the processes of growth and ocular cells differentiation are repeatedly investigated on the model of experimental deprivation myopia in a chicken. Daily intravitreal injection of selective antagonists of serotonin and nicotine exerts restrictive influence on myopia progressing; however, some of them induce negative changes in pigmented retinal epithelium [179].

The obtained data allow authors to make a conclusion that serotonin and acetylcholine exert stimulating influence on processes of growth and ocular cells differentiation, and serotonin and N-cholinoreceptors are included in ocular growth controlling system [60, 179].

* * *

In conclusion, it should be noted that modern ophthalmology improves mainly surgical methods of cataract treatment. Questions concerning etiology and pathogenesis of the given disease are remained without due attention.

However, last year, there appeared a tendency to study fine biochemical and immunohistochemical bases of lens exchange normally and in conditions of cataractogenesis. Consequences of such fundamental approach are data about trophic influence disturbances of the lens, initiating disturbances of different links of cellular metabolism and, consequently, of certain structural transformations of its cell.

Chapter IV

Material and Methods

Material for investigation of the changed lenses due to cataract was obtained during the planned surgical treatment of age cataract in patients at the ages of 60-70.

Controls were 17 lenses of dead young men of 20-30 y.o., obtained by enucleation of eyeballs during 12 hours from the moments of death due to accidents. Enucleation was carried on with the purpose of the planned transplantation of donor cornea.

Investigated material was divided into three groups: first group (control group) – 17 intact lenses; second group – 114 lenses, affected by age cortical cataract; third group – 170 lenses, affected by age nuclear cataract.

Frozen and paraffin sagittal sections of the lens with 15 mcm thickness were treated by the following methods:

1. *Hematoxylin and eosin stain* was used as the general histological stain of the lens [149].
2. With the purpose of histamine-containing structures, identification fresh frozen sections of the lens were treated by *fluorescent-histochemical methods of Cross – Even – Rost* [35]. The method is based on vapor reaction of alpha-orthophaldehyde with histamine, in the course of which fluorescent connections of imidazolylethylamine are formed. Under fluorescence microscope, the formed complex product in large histamine content gives yellow fluorescence, in average–green, in small – blue.
   Lens sections were treated in the preliminary heated chamber by alpha-orthophaldehyde vapors in the thermostat at temperature 100oC

for ten sec. Then sections were placed in another chamber, containing water vapors, at the same temperature for two min. Later sections were dried up in the thermostat at temperature 70oC for five min, after that were contained into polystyrene. Preparations were studied for two hours from the moment of reaction appearance.

3. *Fluorescent-histochemical methods of Falk – Hillarp* [52, 53], based on catecholamines condensation by formaldehyde with 1, 2, 3, 4-terahydroisoquinoline formation, which change as a result into high fluorescent 3, 2-dihydroconnections of isoquinoline. These products form the fluorescent complex, giving bright green fluorescence. Carbolines, which in similar reactions form serotonin, give white and yellow fluorescence. Fluorescent-histochemical methods in modification of M. Krokhina differ from original methods of Falk by fresh frozen sections drying up in air without freeze-drying.

4. Quantative bioamines concentrations in various lens structures were estimated by means of *cytospectrofluorometry* [90, 187]. For this, the nozzle FMEL-1A in output voltage 900V was set on the fluorescent microscope LYUMAM-4. The light from the fluorescent preparation, hitting the add-on device, passed through the special orifice-sonde with diameter 0.5 mm, cutting out an area in the preparation plane, light from which hit the interference color filter with the certain wave length.

For fluorescence intensity measuring of histamine, the color filter №7 with wave length 515 nm was applied, for fluorescence intensity determining of catecholamines the color filter №6 with wave length 480 nm was used, for serotonin - №8 with wave length 525 nm. Fluorescence intensity measurement was carried out in units of fluorescence (conventional units according to the scale of registering apparatus- amplifier) in ten fields of vision by means of objective 40, ocular 15.

5. *Complex of immunohistochemical reactions* with monoclonal antibodies to: neuronspecific enolase (NSE), protein S-100 (S-100), vimetin (Vim), α-smooth muscular actin (α-SMA) and pancytokeratin (EMA).

Material, obtained in the course of planned surgical extraction of age cataract or intracapsular extraction of the lens, was fixed in 10% neutral formaldehyde solution. Material was dehydrated in ethanol of gradually increasing concentration and put in paraffin.

Lens sections with 15mcm thickness were obtained on paraffin microtome MPS-2. After removing of paraffin and dehydration in ethanol of decreasing concentration, lens sections were imbedded in regenerating citrate buffer (pH 6.0), then high-temperature treatment by heating on water bath at 90-95°C for 30 min with the purpose of demasking of required antigens in tissues was carried on.

After inhibiting of endogenous peroxidase by 3% hydrogen peroxide solution on methanol, immunohistochemical reaction was carried on by three-stage indirect immunoenzymatic analysis method with primary monoclonal antibodies using the following antigenic markers: neuronspecific enolase (NSE), protein S-100 (S-100), vimetin (Vim), α-smooth muscular actin (α-SMA) and pancytokeratin (EMA).

The mentioned primary monoclonal antibodies were used in dilutions according to the enclosed recommendations of the firm-producer "Novocastra" (Great Britain) – NSE (1:50), S-100 (1:50), Vim (1:100), α-SMA (1:50), EMA (1:200).

Results' visualization was carried out by peroxidase activity revealing, by its histochemical revealing with chromogen-substrate mixture using on the base of 3-amino-9-ethylcarbazole. Expression specificity of the required antigen in the experimental samples was confirmed by its absence in control sections, untreated by primary monoclonal antibodies. On the final stage, the sections were stained by hematoxylin and concluded into glycerin- gelatin.

6. *Statistic processing.* The mathematical analysis of results of morphological, clinical and experimental sections of research with the subsequent statistical processing of the received data. Statistical reliability of results is defined by nonparametric criterion – the Mann-Whitney U-test [8, 70].

Chapter V

Results

5.1. Common Morphological Changes in the Lens in Conditions of Different Kinds Formation of Age Cataract in a Human Being

Clinical manifestations of the cortical and nuclear kinds of age cataract have no great resemblance. They resemble each other only in time of their origin (at the age over 60) and in progressing of visual acuity decrease due to gradual loss of lens transparence. Many important clinical distinctions of cortical and nuclear kinds of age cataract is of great interest.

Modern ophthalmology distinguishes the following peculiarities of clinical course of the given kinds of age cataract: primary localization opacity (in cortical and nuclear parts of a lens), presence and absence of dehydration signs of the lens (formation of water fissures, vacuoles or lens thickening without dehydration signs), different colors of opacity (gray or brown, respectively).

Light microscopy and general histological hematoxylin and eosin stain of saggital paraffin sections of changed lenses due to cataract also allow revealing morphological distinctions of different kinds of age cataract.

The intact human lens is located in the posterior chamber of the eye, isolated from other membranes by the ocular capsule, and doesn't contain nerves, vessels (Pic. 1). The equator and two poles – anterior and posterior – are distinguished. Along the equator, the lens is symbolically divided into the anterior and posterior surfaces. Histologically, the intact lens consists of the capsule, its epithelium and lens cells-fibers (Pic. 3, 4). The internal surface of the anterior capsule is covered with lens epithelial cells – this is a layer of anterior epithelial cells, so-called lens anterior epithelium. In the region of lens, equator covering with epithelial cells is finished. At the equator, epithelial cells of lens are subjected to mitotic division (Pic. 2, 4) and acquire elongated form, transforming into young lens cells-fibers, which forms superficial cortical layer of the lens (Pic. 4). Lens cells-fibers, as anterior epithelial cells, possess the nucleus and large part of common cytoplasmatic organelles. In cells-fibers transformation into lens fibers, their nuclear chromatin and nuclei disappear. In the course of further differentiation, gradual cytomembranes loss takes place, as a result of which compact, dense nucleus of the lens, having no cellular structure, is formed. In *the cortical variant* of age cataract, one can see: distinct dehydration of the cortical part of the lens, lens cells-fibers dissociation, sphenoid spaces, filled with detritus and vacuoles, besides, on the border of the cortical and nuclear parts the zone of intensive vacuolization is formed (Pic. 5). The nuclear part of the lens is compressed by hydrated cortical masses but has no structural deviation from a norm. In *the nuclear variant* formation of age cataract, general histological hematoxylin and eosin stain of sections reveals in the region of the lens nucleus the accumulation of homogenous material, which increases it in size, resulting in unchanged cortical layer compression (Pic. 6).

* * *

Thus, the above-mentioned facts, distinguishing morphological process of cortical and nuclear kinds formation of age cataract, are the evidence that the influence of such a causative agent as age on the lens can be realized through quite different pathogenetic mechanisms, further resulting in formation of this or that kind of age cataract.

5.2. Bioamines Profile of the Lens in Conditions of Different Kinds Formation of Age Cataract in a Human Being

Biogenic amines, being universal hormones-mediators of nervous, endocrine and immune systems, take part in great number of regulatory processes in the body; at the same time, their participation in regulation of various structural and functional characteristics of the lens is practically not investigated. In spite of considerable number of works concerned with pathogenesis studying and cataract therapy, morphological aspects of its origin and the possible role of humoral disturbances in development of this disease remain a little investigated.

In fluorescent microscopy of *intact lens sections* (Pic. 7), treated with α-orthophaldehyde vapors according to Cross's method [35], the lens nucleus is well visualized; its fluorescence is highly marked, has emerald-green color and doesn't become dim for a long time. Fluorescence of the intact lens nucleus is determined by flash of its central parts, magnitude of which according to spectrofluorimetry averages 0.0595 ± 0.0014 mv (Pic. 8). Fluorescence in the given region may be characterized as the most intensive and bright on the section.

In the region of the intact lens cortex, fluorescence is less marked; it also has emerald-green color but becomes dim faster. Fluorescence of the intact lens cortex is determined according to cytoplasmic fluorescence of lens fibers, forming its cortex and averages 0.0511 ± 0.0024 mv (Pic. 8). Cellular membranes of lens fibers are not revealed.

In age *cortical cataract* histamine level is subjected to considerable changes (Pic. 8). According to data of spectrofluorimetry, histamine concentration in the region of the lens cortex increases more than 42.9% (Pic. 8), which averages 0.0730 ± 0.0029 mv ($P<0.05$). Fluorescence of the cortical and nuclear parts is considerably increased, acquires yellow-green tone and doesn't become dim for a long time. Cytomembranes are not revealed either. Fluorescence in the lens nuclear part, as before, remains the most intensive, bright on the section 0.0899 ± 0.0028 mv, $P<0.05$ and exceeds histamine level in the intact lens nucleus more than 51%.

Other tendency is browsing in conditions of age *nuclear cataract* formation (Pic. 8). Fluorescence of lens sections is moderately marked, has emerald-green color, and visually fluorescence intensity of the cortical and nuclear parts of the lens is practically the same. Thus, in the lens cortical part, histamine concentration is practically no different from a norm's indices 0.0525 ± 0.0041 mv ($P<0.01$), histamine level increases only more than 2.7%, in the lens nuclear part histamine level increases more than 7% and averages 0.0637 ± 0.0034 mv, $P<0.05$ (Pic. 8).

Fluorescence of *the intact lens*, stained according to Falk – Hillarp's method [52, 53] with the purpose of selective investigation of levels of catecholamines and serotonin in it, is moderately marked and has emerald-green color. Visually, fluorescence intensity of lens nucleus exceeds, to a certain extent, fluorescence in its cortical part. According to data of spectrofluorimetry (Pic. 8), catecholamines level in the cortical and nuclear parts of the intact lens is practically the same (0.008±0.0005 mv and 0.0077±0.0005 mv, respectively). It is revealed that serotonin concentration in the lens nuclear part (0.0238±0.0019 mv) exceeds its level in the cortical part (0.0175±0.0004 mv).

In age *cortical cataract* formation, considerable serotonin increase both in the cortical part of the lens (by 1.5 times) and in the nuclear one (by 2.2 times) as well as marked increase of catecholamines concentration in the cortical part of the lens more than 27.5%, in the nuclear one – 57.1%, are revealed.

The nuclear variant development in age cataract is accompanied by sharp (by 3.5 times) serotonin concentration increase in the nuclear part of the lens (Pic. 8), serotonin level in the cortical part is also considerably increased (by three times). Catecholamines level change is also considerable. Catecholamines concentration in the nuclear part of the lens increases by 1.9 times, in its cortical part by 1.5 times.

Comparative analysis carrying on of bioamines state of the lens normally and in different kinds formation of age cataract reveals an interesting regularity (Pic. 8).

In cortical cataract formation, histamine level in the lens increases more than 47%. Considerable increase of serotonin level in the lens more than 93% and marked catecholamines concentration increase (more than 42%) are also revealed.

Other tendency is browsing in nuclear cataract formation. This variant development of age cataract is accompanied by sharp (by 3.3 times) serotonin concentration increase in the lens. Catecholamines level increases more than 70%. Histamine concentration in the lens is practically no different from a norm's indices, increase averages only 4.9%.

While bioamines profile composing of the lens normally and in different kinds of age cataract (Pic. 8), the following is revealed:

- in the cortical variant formation, the synchronous considerable increase of concentrations of all the studied bioamines takes place;
- in consideration of bioamines profile of nuclear cataract, the considerable levels increase of serotonin and catecholamines only is revealed. Histamine concentration is practically no different from a norm's indices.

If concentration of studied bioamines in the intact lens is taken as 100%, conditions of bioamines supply of the lens, necessary for different kinds of formations of age cataract, can be presented as follows (Pic. 8):

- ✓ for the cortical kind formation of cataract, the necessary condition is the synchronous considerable increase of concentrations of histamine, serotonin and catecholamines in the lens;
- ✓ for the nuclear kind formation of cataract, the necessary condition is the synchronous considerable concentrations increase of serotonin and catecholamines only. Histamine level remains practically unchanged.

* * *

Thus, the given results of fluorescence-and-histochemical investigation of the lens show considerable plasticity and fundamental distinctions in bioamines supply of formation processes of the cortical and nuclear kinds of age cataract in a human being.

5.3. Immunohistochemical Investigation of Lens Cells in Conditions of Different Kinds Formation of Age Cataract in a Human Being

In carrying on immunohistochemical reactions with monoclonal antibodies to neuronspecific enolase (NSE), protein S-100 (S-100), vimentin (Vim), α-smooth muscular actin (α-SMA), pancytokeratin (EMA) in all parts of the human intact lens the specific staining didn't occur, and structural deviations from a norm were not revealed (Pic. 9).

Immunohistochemical stain and light microscopy of paraffin sections of changed lenses due to cataract reveal sufficiently distinct morphological distinctions of different kinds of age cataract.

In cortical cataract, the positive reaction of the same type for antibodies to protein S-100 (Pic. 10), Vim (Pic. 11) and NSE (Pic. 12), more marked for antibodies to NSE, is immunohistochemically revealed. Cells of lens anterior epithelium show moderately marked positive stain.

In lens cortical layer between swollen lens cells-fibers, the fissures and sphenoid spaces, filled with detritus and single vacuoles, are revealed, in the region of formation of which there is the intensive reaction for the mentioned indices.

It is important to note that intensive stain for the given antibodies, possessing also intracellular localization in cytoplasm of several cells-fibers in the form of granules, evenly distributed along the whole cytoplasm, is revealed (Pic. 16).

On the border of cortical and nuclear layers of the lens the distinct zone of intensive vacuolization is examined, in which slight positive reaction to NSE, S-100 and Vim is also revealed. It is important to note that in the lens nuclear part, the mentioned antibodies don't give specific stain. In immunohistochemical investigation with monoclonal antibodies using the negative reaction both in the cortical and nuclear parts of the lens to α-SMA (Pic. 13) and EMA is revealed.

In age, nuclear cataract development in the lens nuclear part the positive reaction for monoclonal antibodies to α-SMA (Pic. 14) and EMA (Pic. 15), which has marked focal character, is immunohistochemically revealed.

For all that, it is revealed that anterior epithelial cells and lens cell-fibers, forming cortical layer of the lens, don't show specific staining to α-SMA and EMA. In monoclonal antibodies using to NSE, S-100 and Vim the lens sections in conditions of nuclear cataract don't show specific staining.

While analyzing the carried on investigation, it can be noted that the human intact lens doesn't show specific staining to the applied in the given investigation monoclonal antibodies (NSE, S-100, Vim, α-SMA, EMA) and, consequently, in the intact lens, the immunohistochemical marks on the main types of body's tissues are lacking.

In age, cortical cataract development in the lens the appearing of positive reaction to certain monoclonal bodies (NSE, S-100 and Vim) can be noted, the region of specific reaction appearance being lined only in the lens cortical part.

In the nuclear variant formation of age cataract, the specific staining is revealed only in the lens nuclear part. Positive reaction appearance is connected with the using of monoclonal antibodies to α-SMA and EMA.

Preliminary analysis of data allows speaking about the revealing of certain transformation regularities of lenticular cellular phenotypes, taking place at its pathological aging.

* * *

Thus, the results of carried on immunohistochemical investigation show considerable plasticity of lens cellular phenotypes normally and in its age opacity, showing that formation of a certain kind of human age cataract depends on changes by lens cells of their phenotypical characteristics, specific molecular mechanisms of which have to be studied more.

Chapter VI

Results' Discussion

6.1. The Analysis of Common Morphological Changes of the Lens in Conditions of Different Kinds Formation of Age Cataract in a Human Being

At present, many aspects of structure, functions and intracellular interactions of ocular tissues are investigated. The interest in these questions is inspired in connection with the presence of large number of diseases, for which practical medicine has no reliable methods of prophylaxis and treatment. Cataract can be served as an example of such disease, as nowadays there is no conservative method able to treat or stop the process of lens opacity for a long period of time.

Cataract is used to consider as a multifactor, polyetiological disease – senile, traumatic, radial, etc. [24, 50].

However, the above-mentioned factors are only the varieties of injuring effects and symbolic notation of changed conditions of organism's vital activity in the whole and the lens in particular. The true cause, initiating catarctogenesis process, undoubtedly, is more delicately organized. And, probably, it should be found in such fields of natural science as membraneology, molecular biology, biochemistry and biophysics.

Last year, there appeared a tendency to study the exchange processes of the lens from the point of view of structural and functional organization of membranes of its cells and fibers – receptors supply, calcium permeability and mechanisms of its regulation, regularity of spatial organization of membranes [30, 32, 45, 46, 74, 113, 126, 134, 140, 146, 152, 200].

The given data about pathological morphological changes of the lens in cataractogenesis process fully agree with data of the present investigation and are the evidence of existence of important distinctions in pathogenesis of different kinds of age cataract.

For example, since the time of early Chinese and early Greek medicine, it has been known about division of cataract into two main kinds – "gray" and "brown." Discoveries made by Antoin Metr-Jan and Jack Daviel in the beginning of XVII century, served the basis for determining of opacity localization and were reflected in new terminology – the above-mentioned kinds of age cataract we began call "cortical" and "nuclear." Clinical manifestations of the cortical and nuclear kinds of age cataract have no great resemblance. They resemble each other only in the time of their origin (age over 60) and also in progressing decrease of visual acuity due to gradual lens transparence loss. Much more important distinctions are of interest, to which the primary opacity localization, the presence and absence of lens hydration signs, various color of opacity can be referred.

Pathological morphology of the cortical kind of age cataract is characterized by appearance in the lens cortical part of water fissures, dissociation of cortex, humor, accumulating in extracellular space. Later, there occurs opacity of radial water fissures and formation of larger pin-shaped and sphenoid opacity, which gradually move in direction of the lens anterior and posterior capsule, and on the stage of mature cortical cataract, the whole cortex is subjected to opacity, acquiring grayish-white color ("gray" cataract). In rare cases due to lyze of opacity diluted cortical masses of the lens and its nucleus, the visual function restoration can even take place. This phenomenon is called spontaneous resorption of age cortical cataract in the course of its hypermaturing (Morgagnian cataract). Such outcome is characteristic only of the cortical kind of age cataract. Described to nowadays morphological changes, characteristic to age cortical cataract, gave grounds to new change of terminology and introduction of the term "extracellular cataract" [78].

In the nuclear kind formation of age cataract, the primary opacity appears in internal embryonic nucleus of the lens and in cellular cytoplasm of the lens nucleus, spreading then on all parts of the mature nucleus. Opacity has reddish or brownish color ("brown" cataract), has homogeneous character and is distributed diffusively [141]. In the hypermaturing of age nuclear cataract, vice versa, excessive thickening of the whole lens substance is observed and "hard," "brown" cataract is formed. Such outcome is characteristic only of the nuclear kind of age cataract. The thickening predominance of fibers over their lyze differs nuclear age cataract from the cortical one.

Besides the investigation of ultrastructural disturbances of the lens with scanning electronic microscopy, applying in conditions of nuclear cataract development in old patients revealed in the lens the formation of regions of its "globular degeneration" [62]. They consist of spherical protein globules (multilamellar bodies, MLBs) with diameter from 1 to 2 mcm, covered with double-layer lipid membrane and are able to decrease optical transmission more than 65% [62].

In cytoplasm of lens epithelial cells and lens cells-fibers, the granules of glycogen with size 25-35 nm are revealed [121]. It is important to note that the described pathological changes of the lens were not described in patients with the cortical kind of age cataract [34, 57].

The revealed morphological peculiarities of the nuclear kind formation of age cataract are the grounds for terminology's change, reflecting the level of modern knowledge and introduction of the term "intracellular cataract" [78].

The existence of important pathogenetic distinctions of age cortical and nuclear cataract is confirmed by many experimental models of cataractogenesis, the result of which is specific kind modeling of opacity.

Thus, with the purpose of the cortical kind reconstruction of cataract, the model of cataractogenesis by applying of lens incubation in calcium-saturated medium is suggested [113]. With the purpose of the nuclear kind modeling of cataract, the lens injury with applying of hyperbaric oxygenation is suggested [56], as hyperbaric oxygenation, according to data of electronic microscopy, initiates fine, but important morphological changes of cytoplasmatic structures by the type of its reorganization in mild oxygenation, which is characteristic of age nuclear cataract.

The models of cataractogenesis of vertebrate animals in vitro by means of intact lenses' cultivation with unremoved capsule in nutrient medium with addition of cataractogenic agents (calcium chloride and hydrogen peroxide) for initiation of the cortical and nuclear kinds formation of cataract, respectively, are of common knowledge.

* * *

Thus, the data given above about the existence of important morphological distinctions of processes formation of the cortical and nuclear kinds of age cataract are the evidence that effect of such a causative agent as age on the lens can be realized through quite different pathogenesis, resulting in future in formation of this or that kind of age-related cataract.

6.2. The Analysis of Bioamines Supply of Processes Formation of Different Kinds Formation of Age Cataract in a Human Being

The humoral system exerts considerable influence on functioning regulation of lens cells. In particular, it is shown that both excess and lack of some hormones, for example, glycocorticoids, is accompanied by lens opacity – Itsenko-Kushing's disease, Simmond's disease [89]. The importance of the humoral system in various characteristics regulation of lens cells is confirmed by the fact that these cells express large amount of receptors: H_1-histamino – [32, 146]; M_1-cholino – [45], M_3-cholino – [31]; P_2U-, P_2Y_2-purino – and $α_1$-adreno – receptors [30]; mineralocorticoidal receptors [126]; glucocorticoidal receptors [74]; receptors to sex hormones – estrogenic, progesteronic, androgenic [72, 73, 198]; as well as signal receptors of the epidermal growth factor [195] and many others [143, 195].

One of the least investigated aspects of humoral regulation of lens cells functioning is their biogenic amines supply. Modern data, characterizing the role of histamine in exchange processes of the lens, are the evidence of both its participation in the course of pathological process [113] and importance of histamine properties directed to participation in the process of cellular division [118, 200] and also to the fight with cataractogenesis [156].

Manifestations, connected with realization of physiological [120] and pathological [25-28, 63] effects of catecholamines in ocular tissues, are also important and many sided. Data, obtained in the studying of serotonin effects, allowed concluding that serotonin exerts the stimulating influence on the processes of growth and differentiation of eyeball's cells, and serotonin receptors are included in the growth regulation system of the eye [60, 179].

However, increased concentration of serotonin initiates important pathological effects (development change of retinal amacrine cells, level increase of intraocular pressure, constriction of the pupil and blood vessels of the eye) able to initiate rough dystrophic changes [60].

Besides, both marked synergism of physiological and pathological effects of biogenic amines and complex competitive interactions between them were revealed and repeatedly studied [111, 176]. The studying of the possible role of biogenic amines is especially actual, if taking into account the already-described role of histamine in transport regulation of calcium ions through cellular membranes, the excess of which in lens cells is known to be able to initiate the development of one of the cataract's form [113].

It is proved [200] that epithelium and fibers of the intact lens have very low calcium permeability; however, even small exceeding of normal calcium level in lens cells initiates content increase calcium-mobilizing agonists (histamine, ATP, carbachol, sulfur) in them, which supports the work of calcium channels. According to Williams M.R. et al. (2001) [200], agonists (histamine, ATP, carbachol, sulfur) and antagonists of calcium channels, the system of which support the signal system for calcium overload prevention in the lens, are kept in the lens intracellular. The revealed in luminescent-histochemical part of the given investigation fact of considerable increase level of histamine in age cortical cataract formation allows suggesting that the failure in the work of the mentioned signal system has supreme significance for formation of just the cortical kind of cataract.

Comparative analysis of bioamines profile of the lens revealed that in the cortical kind formation of age cataract, the synchronous considerable concentration increase of histamine (more than 47%), serotonin (more than 93%) as well as the marked increase of catecholamines concentration (more than 42%) in the lens take place. In consideration of bioamines profile of nuclear cataract, the considerable increase of serotonin level (by 3.3 times) and marked increase of catecholamines concentration (more than 70%), especially in the nuclear part, were revealed. For all that, histamine level is practically no different from indices of a norm (increase averaged only 4.9%).

*** * ***

Thus, the revealed by the given investigation fundamental distinctions of neuromediator supply of formation processes of age cortical and nuclear cataract are the evidence of various pathogenesis existence, resulting in various types of neurodystrophic process in the human lens.

6.3. The Analysis of Phenotypical Characteristics of Lens Cells in Conditions of Different Kinds of Formation of Age Cataract in a Human Being

Modern experimental medicine has numerous evidences of importance of phenotypical characteristics of tissue for keeping its function; however, there is only scanty information about lens cellular phenotype change in conditions of its pathology. From literary sources, it is known that in conditions of different kinds formation of cataract in a human being, the positive reactions of lens cells to vimentin were revealed; in this connection, the authors advanced the supposition about lens epithelial cells transformation into mesenchymal in the course of cataractogenesis [183]. On cellular culture of laboratory animals, it shown that in conditions of experimental injury lens cells are subjected to transformation into myofibroblasts, positive to the established marker of this process [154].

The above-mentioned investigations touch upon the fundamental problem of cells phenotype transformation in different conditions and show the possibility of change by lens cells of their phenotypical characteristics in conditions of cataractogenesis.

While analyzing the results of immunohistochemical part of the present investigation, it is necessary to note that the human intact lens doesn't manifest specific staining to the applied monoclonal antibodies (NSE, protein S-100, Vim, α-SMA, EMA) and, consequently, immunohistochemical marks to the main types of body's tissues are lacking in the human intact lens.

The cause of this is, probably, the hematoophthalmological barrier, the presence of which supplies the eyeball's structures with the status of post-barrier ones. It is known that age diseases formation of the organ of vision, including also age cataract, are accompanied by permeability change of hematoophthalmological barrier [172], the disturbance of which is closely interconnected with the described in the present investigation change of neuromediator control (bioamines profile) of a cell.

In development of human age cortical cataract, the appearance of positive reaction to certain monoclonal antibodies (NSE, protein S-100 and Vim) is revealed for all that the zone of specific reaction appearance is lined just with lens cortical part.

In formation of the nuclear kind of age cataract, the specific staining is revealed only in the lens nuclear part and is connected with monoclonal antibodies using to α-smooth muscular actin (α-SMA) and pancytokeratin (EMA).

The analysis of the obtained data allows speaking about the revealing of certain regularities of phenotype transformation of lens cells occurring in its pathological aging. Mesenchymal-neuroectodermal direction of phenotype transformation of lens cells is characteristic to the formation of the cortical kind of age cataract. For all that, the appearance of the nuclear kind of age cataract is accompanied by formation of myoepithelial direction.

It is evident that lens epithelial cells in formation of age cortical cataract are in conditions, which contribute their further accelerated differentiation, "evolution," "acquiring of specialization signs," "complication of structure" [186, 194], which means differentiation of biochemical components of a cell (bioamines profile) and also differentiation of cellular organelles (expression of specific proteins).

In appearance of age, nuclear cataract lens epithelial cells are in the influence of the factors, contributing to "involution," "cell's return to ontogenetic past," "cell's acquiring of embryonic signs," "back cell's development," " loss of specialization signs," "dedifferentiation" [186, 194], which means differentiation of both biochemical components of a cell (bioamines profile), and de-differentiation of cellular organelles (expression of specific proteins).

The results of the present investigation agree with data of many investigators, repeatedly speaking about the presence of phenomenon as cellular phenotype transformation under the influence of a number of external and internal factors [9, 40, 154, 183]. More often, they speak about the transition of cellular epithelial phenotype into mesenchymal, so-called epithelial-mesenchymal transition, which is considered the fundamental process, controlling morphogenesis in multicellular organism [185].

The close connection of phenotype of lens cells and ability to perform functions specific for it is of great importance for practical ophthalmology, too, as the change of phenotypical characteristics of lens cells is inevitably connected with structural reorganization of these cells, and, consequently, with the change of their optical properties, which are clinically manifested by lens opacity disturbance in age cataract formation.

* * *

Thus, it is revealed that formation of the certain kind of age-related cataract in a human being depends on lens cells' change of their phenotypical characteristics.

Conclusion

Considerable morphological distinctions of formation processes of the cortical and nuclear kinds of age cataract are the evidence that the influence of such a causative agent as age on the human lens can be realized through quite different pathogenesis, resulting further in formation of this or that kind of age-related cataract.

Human lens epithelial cells normally and in its age opacity contain histamine, serotonin and catecholamines. Conditions of bioamines supply of formation processes of different kinds of human age cataract are not the same and have fundamental distinctions: the necessary condition for the cortical kind formation is the simultaneous considerable concentration increase of histamine, serotonin and catecholamines in the lens; for the nuclear kind formation, the simultaneous considerable concentration increase of histamine, catecholamines and changes' absence of histamine concentration are necessary.

The human intact lens doesn't contain immunohistochemical marks on the main types of tissues of the body. However, its pathological aging is induced by lens cells' change of their phenotypical characteristics and formation of different pathological phenotypes of lens cells, determining formation of the cortical and nuclear kind of human age cataract.

By the results of the present investigation, the necessity of differentiated approach of formation of preventive and therapeutic measures of human age-related cataract, depending on its specific kind, are pathogenetically proved.

Appendix

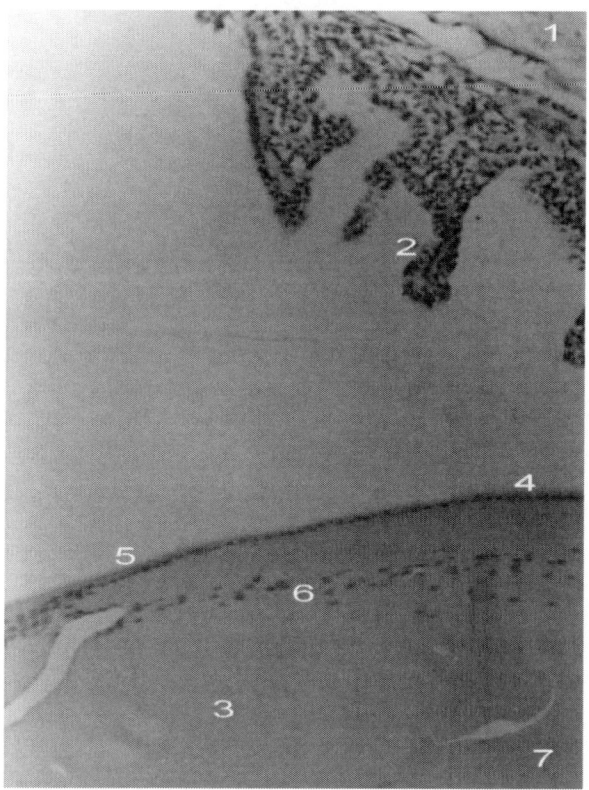

Picture 1. Microscopic structure of eyeball. Sagittal section. Staining by hematoxylin-eosin. Magn.: obj. 20, oc. 15. 1 – sclera, 2 – **ciliary body's processes**, 3 – cortex of lens, 4 – central part of anterior epithelium of lens, 5 – equatorial part of anterior epithelium of lens (a growth zone), 6 – cells-fibers forming a cortex of lens, 7–nucleus of lens.

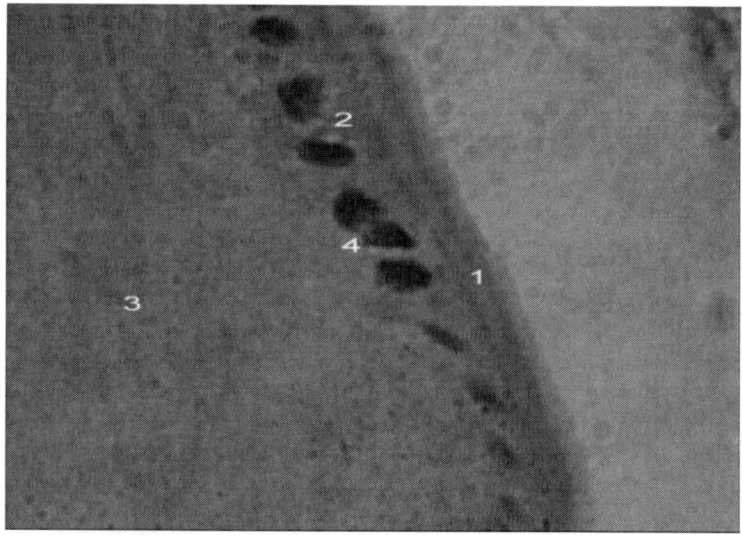

Picture 2. Mitotic activity of equatorial epithelial cells of intact lens in the zone of its growth. Staining by ferrous hematoxylin. Magn.: obj. 90, oc. 15. 1 – capsule of lens, 2 – equatorial cells of anterior epithelium of lens, 3 – peripheral parts of lenticular cells-fibers, 4 – mitotic division of the lens equatorial epithelial cell.

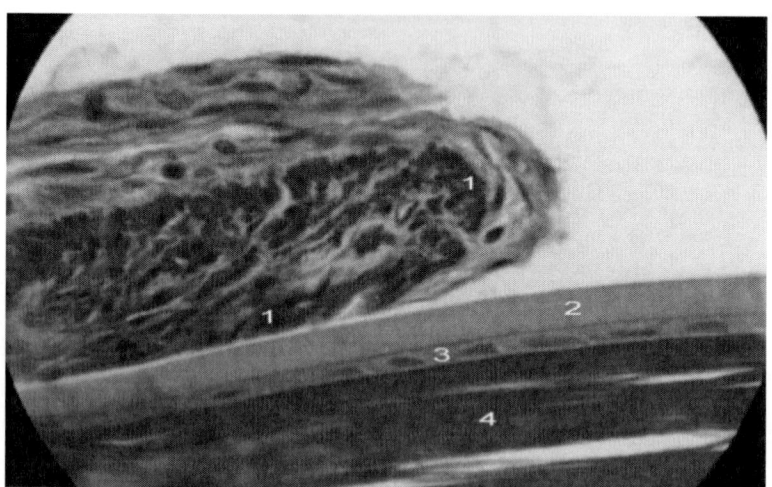

Picture 3. Sagittal section of intact lens. Staining by hematoxylin-eosin. Magn.: obj. 90, oc. 15. 1 – iris, 2 – capsule of lens, 3 – cells of anterior epithelium of lens (the central part), 4 – cells-fibers forming cortex of lens.

Appendix

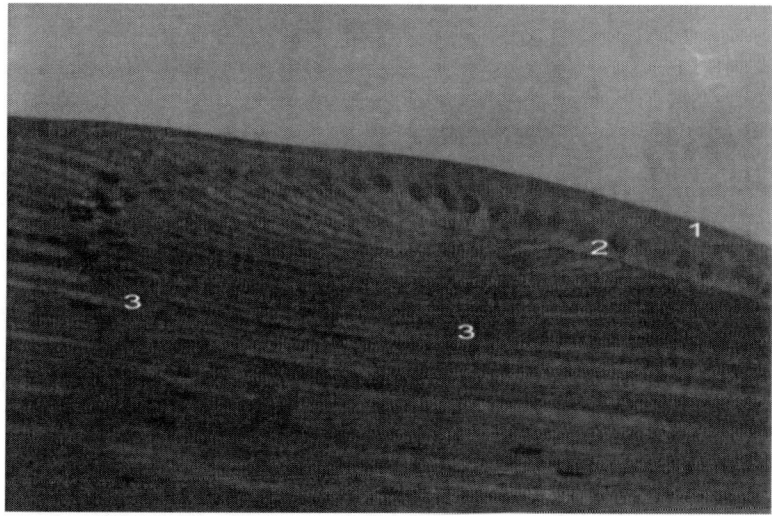

Picture 4. Sagittal section of intact lens. The improved method of common histological stain of lens (Patent of Russian Federation for the invention № 2319132 from 24.08.2005). Magn.: obj. 40, oc. 15. 1 – capsule of lens, 2 – equatorial cells of lens anterior epithelium (the growth zone), 3 – cells-fibers forming cortex of lens.

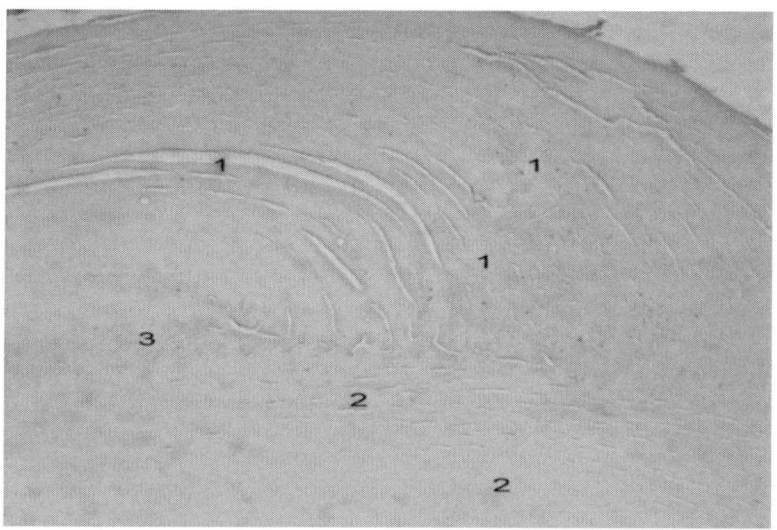

Picture 5. Sagittal section of human lens with age-related cortical cataract. Staining by hematoxylin-eosin. Magn.: obj. 40, oc. 15. 1 – cortex of lens with the hydration signs (the cells-fibers dissociation, the wedge-shaped spaces filled with detritus and vacuoles), 2 – nucleus of lens compressed by hydrated cortical masses, 3 – the zone of vacuolization.

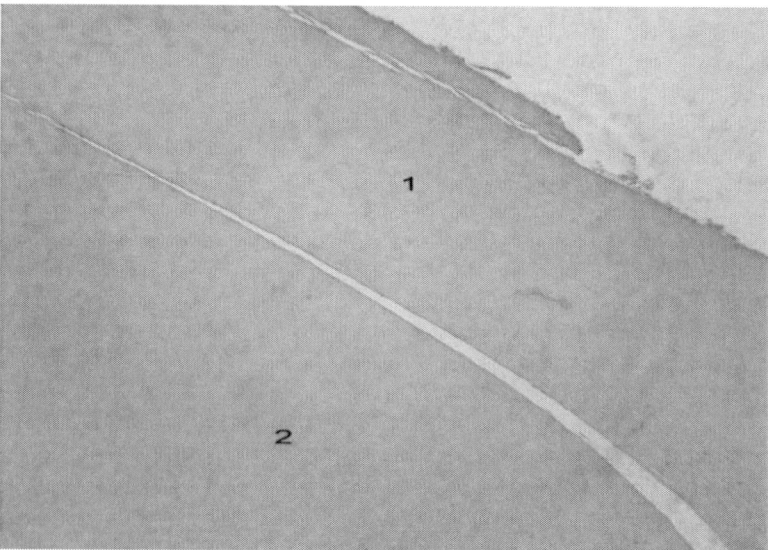

Picture 6. Sagittal section of human lens with age-related nuclear cataract. Staining by hematoxylin-eosin. Magn.: obj. 40, oc. 15. 1 – cortex of lens without hydration signs, 2 – homogenous nucleus of lens increased in volume.

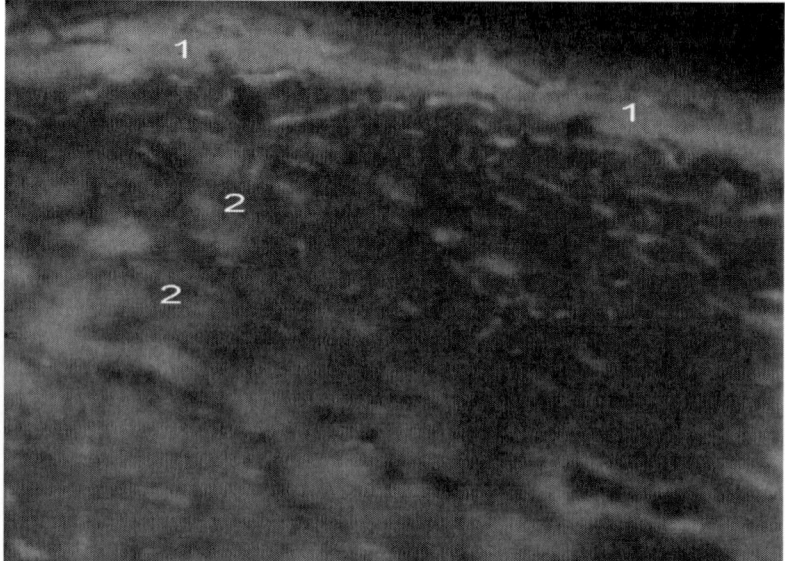

Picture 7. Histamine-containing structures of equatorial part of intact lens. Staining according to the method of Cross – Even – Rost [35]. Magn.: obj. 40, oc. 15. 1 – equatorial cells of anterior epithelium of lens, 2 – cells-fibers forming cortex of lens.

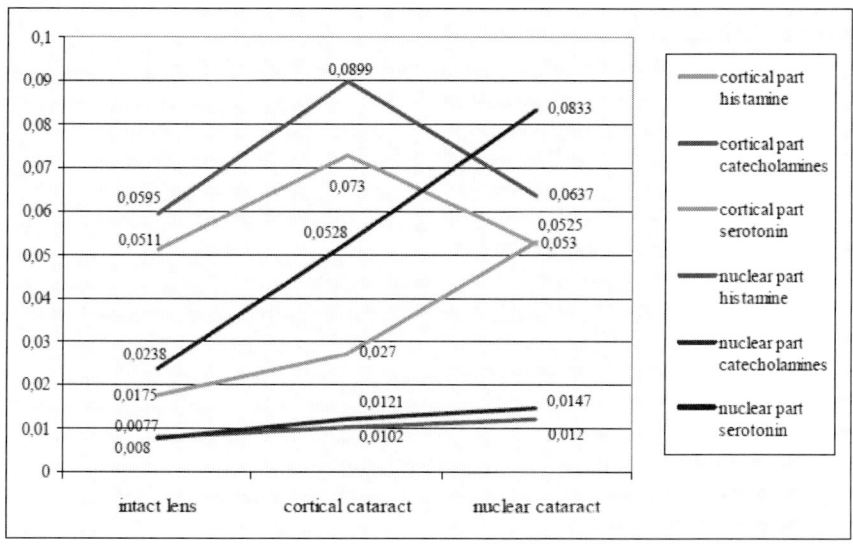

Picture 8. The change of bioamines concentrations (histamine, serotonin, catecholamines) in intact lens and in different kinds of human age cataract.

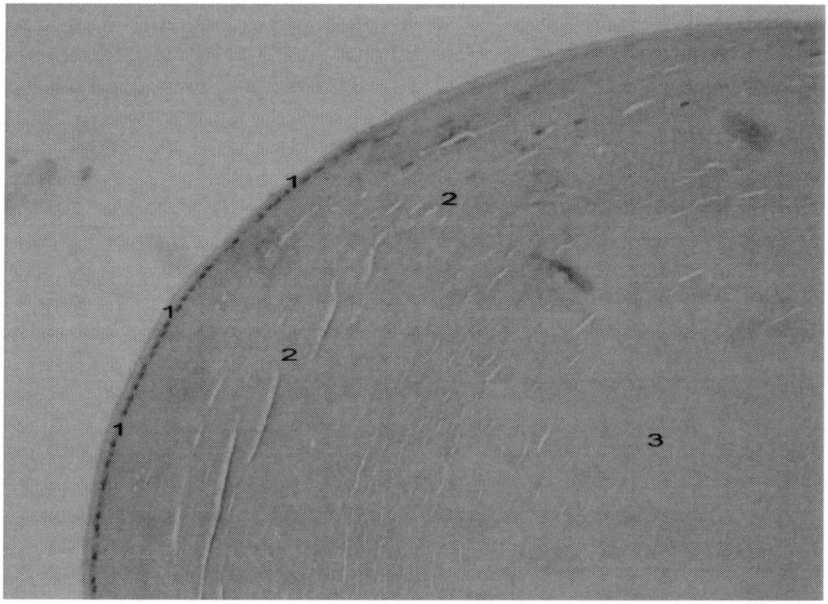

Picture 9. Morphological structure of intact human lens. Staining by hematoxylin-eosin. Magn.: obj. 40, oc. 15. 1 – epithelium of anterior lens capsule, 2 – cortical department of lens, 3 – nuclear department of lens.

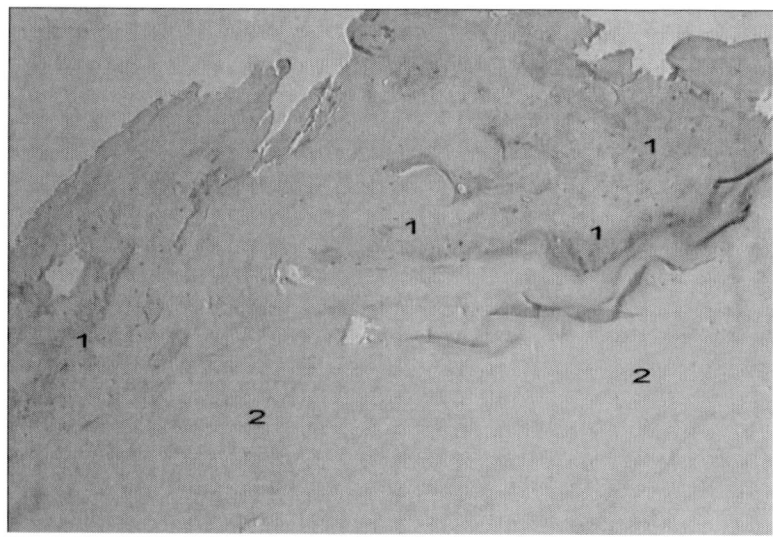

Picture 10. Age-related cortical cataract. Immunohistochemical staining with monoclonal antibodies to protein S-100. Magn.: obj. 40, oc. 15. 1 – S-100-immuno-positive sites of lens cortical department, 2 – S-100-immunonegative sites of lens nuclear department.

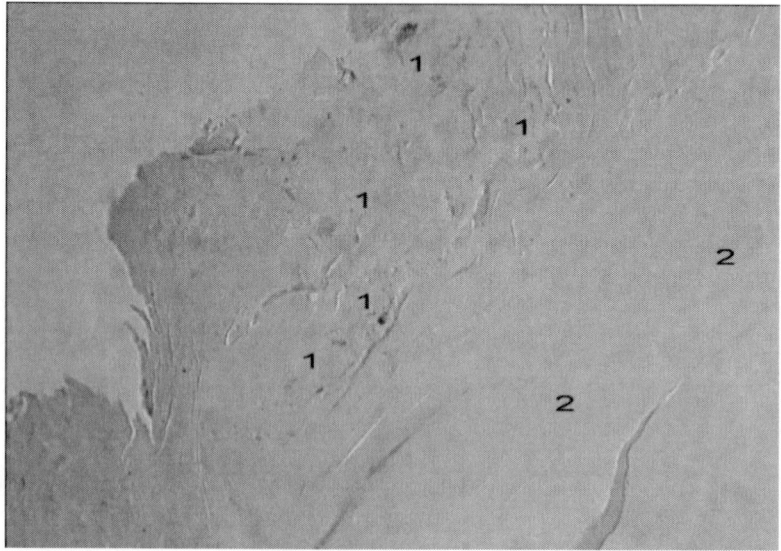

Picture 11. Age-related cortical cataract. Immunohistochemical staining with monoclonal antibodies to Vim. Magn.: obj. 40, oc. 15. 1 – Vim-immunopositive sites of lens cortical department, 2 – Vim-immunonegative sites of lens nuclear department.

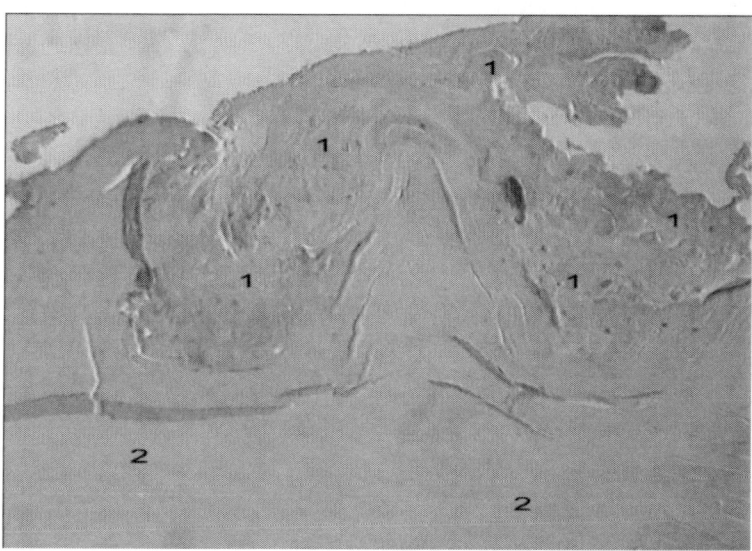

Picture 12. Age-related cortical cataract. Immunohistochemical staining with monoclonal antibodies to NSE. Magn.: obj. 40, oc. 15. 1 – NSE-immunopositive sites of lens cortical department, 2 – NSE-immunonegative sites of lens nuclear department.

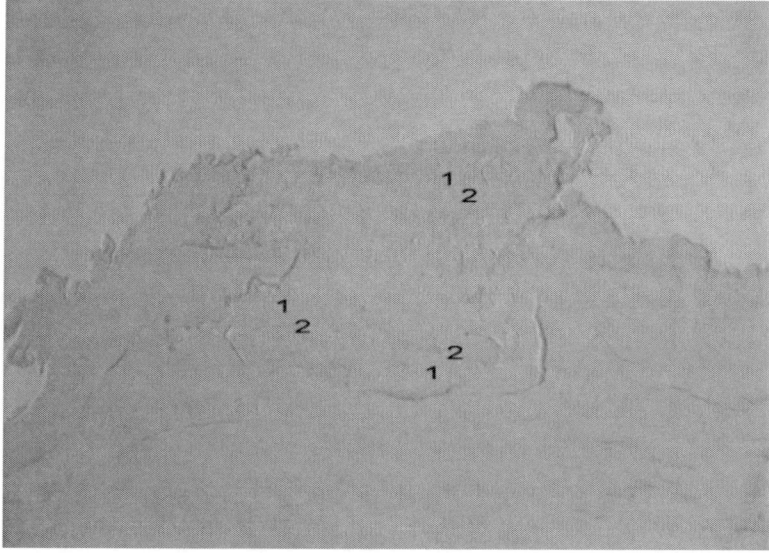

Picture 13. Age-related cortical cataract. Immunohistochemical staining with monoclonal antibodies to α-SMA. Magn.: obj. 40, oc. 15. 1 – pathologically changed sites of lens cortical department, 2 – α-SMA-immunonegative sites of lens cortical department.

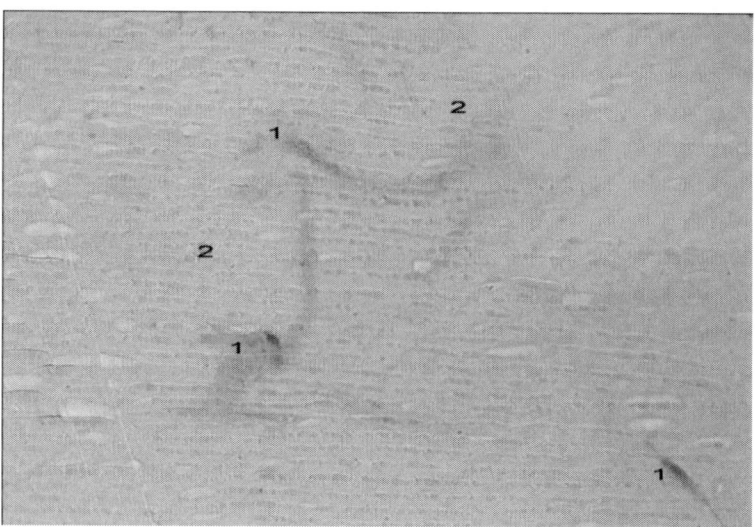

Picture 14. Age-related nuclear cataract. Immunohistochemical staining with monoclonal antibodies to α-SMA. Magn.: obj. 90, oc. 15. 1 – α-SMA-immunopositive sites of lens nuclear department, 2 – α-SMA-immunonegative sites of lens nuclear department.

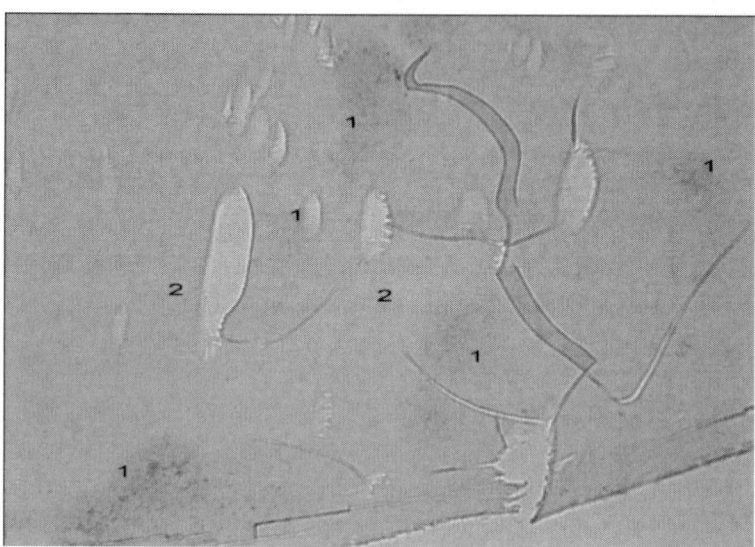

Picture 15. Age-related nuclear cataract. Immunohistochemical staining with monoclonal antibodies to EMA. Magn.: obj. 90, oc. 15. 1 – EMA-immunopositive sites of lens nuclear department, 2 – EMA-immunonegative sites of lens nuclear department.

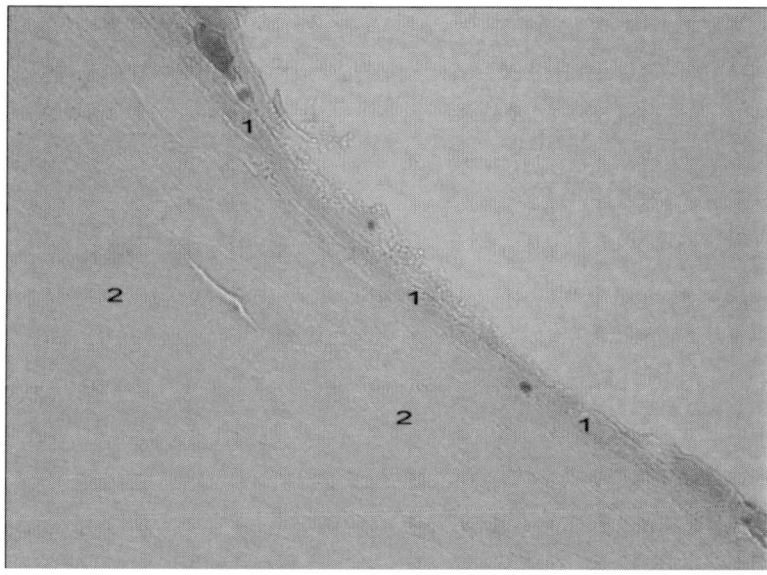

Picture 16. Age-related cortical cataract. Immunohistochemical staining with monoclonal antibodies to NSE. Magn.: obj. 90, oc. 15. 1 – NSE-immunopositive reactions of cytoplasm of the lens cell-fiber, 2 – NSE-immunonegative sites of lens cortical department.

References

[1] Abe H., Honma S., Ohtsu H., Honma K. Circadian rhythms in behavior and clock gene expressions in the brain of mice lacking histidine decarboxylase // *Brain. Res. Mol. Brain. Res.* − 2004. − V.124. − N.2. − P.178-187.

[2] Abe H., Itoh M.T., Miyata M., Shimizu K., Sumi Y. Circadian rhythm of serotonin N-acetyltransferase activity in rat lens // *Exp. Eye Res.* − 2000. − V.70. − N.6. − P.805-808.

[3] Agarkov V.A. Structural and histochemical characteristic of lens in ontogenesis and experimental conditions: *The author's abstract dissertation.* − Omsk, 1973. − 19p.

[4] Aita M. The peptides of the immuno-neuro-endocrine system // *Eur. J. Histochem.* − 1993. − N.37, suppl. − P.10.

[5] Alvarez L.J., Candia O.A., Polikoff L.A. Beta-adrenergic stimulation of Na+-K+-Cl2--cotransport activity in the rabbit lens // *Exp. Eye Res.* − 2003. − V.76. − N.1. − P.61-70.

[6] Alvarez L.J., Turner H.C., Candia O.A., Polikoff L.A. Beta-adrenergic inhibition of rabbit lens anterior-surface K+ conductance // *Curr. Eye Res.* − 2003. − V.26. − N.2. − P.95-105.

[7] Andreev A.N. Studying of relationships of cause and effect of an age cataract with biogeochemical factors: *The author's abstract dissertation.* − Odessa, 1992. −19p.

[8] Avtandilov G.G. Computer microtelephotometria in diagnostics of histocitopathology. − M.:RMAPO, 1996. - 256p.

[9] Bariety J., Hill G.S., Mandet C., Irinopoulou T., Jacquot C., Meyrier A., Bruneval P. Glomerular epithelial-mesenchymal transdifferentiation in pauci-immune crescentic glomerulonephritis//*Nephrol. Dial. Transplant.* − 2003. − V.18. − N.9. − P.1777-1784.

[10] Bochkareva A.A, Bazhenov S.I., Ter-Arutjunova N.A. About the change of epithelium of lens capsules at a senile cataract // *Ophthalmology J.* – 1968. – N.7. – P.499-502.
[11] Bogdanovich U.L. About spontaneous dispersion of senile cataracts // *Ophtalmology J.* – 1966. – N.2. – P.114-118.
[12] Bosco L. The problem of the lens regeneration in anuran amphibian lens // *Acta Embryol. Morphol. Exp.* – 1988. – V.9. – N.l. – P.25-38.
[13] Bosco L., Sciacovelli L., Valle C. Experimental analysis of the lens transdifferention process in anuran amphibian tadpoles // *Acta Embryol. Morphol. Exp.* – 1991. – V.2. – N.l. – P.83-84.
[14] Bosco L., Valle C., Willems D. In vivo and in vitro experimental analysis of the lens regeneration in larval Xenopus laevis // *Dev. Growth a. Differ.* – 1993. – V.35. – N.3. – P.257-270.
[15] Bron A.J., Tripathi R.C., Tripathi B.J. *Wolff□s anatomy of the eye and orbit.* Chapman and Hall. – 1997. – P.734.
[16] Brown N.P., Bron A.J. *Lens disorders: A clinical manual of cataract diagnosis.* – Oxford: Butterworth-Heinemann Ltd., 1996. – 268p.
[17] Bueno J.M., Campbell M.C. Polarization properties of the in vitro old human cristalline lens // *Ophthalmic. Physiol. Opt.* – 2003. – V.23. – N.2. – P.109-118.
[18] Buratto L. *Extracapsular cataract microsurgery and posterior chamber intraocular lenses.* – Milano, 1989. – 756p.
[19] Cammarata P.R., Chu S., Moor A., Wang Z., Yang S.H., Simpkins J.W. Subcellular distribution of native estrogen receptor alpha and beta subtypes in cultured human lens epithelial cells // *Exp. Eye Res.* – 2004. – V.78. – N.4. – P.861-871.
[20] Cammarata P.R., Flynn J., Gottipati S., Chu S., Dimitrijevich S., Younes M., Skliris G., Murphy L.C. Differential expression and comparative subcellular localization of estrogen receptor beta isoforms in virally transformed and normal cultured human lens epithelial cells // *Exp. Eye Res.* – 2005. – V.81. – N.2. – P.165-175.
[21] Candia O.A., Zamudio A.C., Polikoff L.A., Alvarez L.J. Distribution of acetylcholine-sensitive currents around the rabbit crystalline lens // *Exp. Eye Res.* – 2002. – V.74. – N.6. – P.769-776.
[22] Carstens E., Kuenzler N., Handwerker H.O. Activation of neurons in rat trigeminal subnucleus caudalis by different irritant chemicals applied to oral or ocular mucosa // *J. Neurophysiol.* – 1998. – V.80. – N.2. – P.465-492.

[23] Casini P., Cerboni C. Glaucoma e cataratta nella sindrome pseudoesfoliativa // *Boll. Oculist.* – 1993. – V.72. – N.2. – P.333-339.
[24] Cataract // Edited by Z.F. Veselovskoj. – Kiev: Book plus, 2002. – 207p.
[25] Cherickchy L.E. Communication cataractogenesis with pathology vitreous bodies // *Materials of 8th congress of ophthalmologists USSR:* Odessa, 1990. – P.267-268.
[26] Cherickchy L.E. Feature of cataractogenesis in conditions of formation of the complicated cataract//*Ophthalmologic J.* – 1992. – N.1. – P.37-41.
[27] Cherickchy L.E., Maltsev E.V. Etiopathogenesis of complications at a uvea pathology // In the book: "Actual problem of uvea pathology." *Theses of the report of 8th International conference of ophthalmologists:* Odessa, 1993. – P.217.
[28] Cherickchy L.E., Maltsev E.V. Protective organism reactions in pathogenesis of cataracts//*Ophthalmologic J.*–1994. – N.3. – P.161-164.
[29] Churchill G.C., Louis C.F. Ca2+ regulation in differentiating lens cells in culture // *Exp. Eye Res.* – 2002. – V.75. – N.1. – P.77-85.
[30] Churchill G.C., Louis C.F. Stimulation of P2U purinergic or alpha 1A adrenergic receptors mobilizes Ca2+ in lens cells // *Invest. Ophthalmol. Vis. Sci.* – 1997. –V.38. – N.5. – P.855-865.
[31] Collison D.J., Coleman R.A., James R.S., Carey J., Duncan G. Characterization of muscarinic receptors in human lens cells by pharmacologic and molecular techniques//*Invest. Ophthalmol. Vis. Sci.* – 2000. – V.41. – N.9. – P.2633-2241.
[32] Collison D.J., Duncan G. Regional differences in functional receptor distribution and calcium mobilization in the intact human lens // *Invest. Ophthalmol. Vis. Sci.* – 2001. –V.42. – N.10. – P.2355-2363.
[33] Collison D.J., Wang L., Wormstone I.M., Duncan G. Spatial characteristics of receptor-induced calcium signaling in human lens capsular bags // *Invest. Ophthalmol. Vis. Sci.* – 2004. –V.45. – N.1. – P.200-205.
[34] Costello M.J., Oliver T.N., Cobo L.M. Cellular architecture in age-related human nuclear cataracts // *Invest. Ophthalmol. Vis. Sci.* – 1992. – V.33. – N.11. – P.3209-3227.
[35] Cross S.A., Even S.W., Rost F.W. A study of methods available for cyto-chemical localization of histamine by fluorescence induced with orthophtaldehyde or acetaldehyde // *Histochem. J.* – 1971. – V.3 – N.6. – P.471-476.

[36] Cruickshanks K.J. Sunlight exposure and risk of lens opacities in a population-based study // *Arch. Ophthal.* – 1998. – V.116. – N.12. – P.1666.
[37] Cruickshanks K.J., Klein B., Klein R. Ultraviolet light exposure and lens opacities: the Beaver Dam eye study // *Am. J. Public Health.* – 1992. – V.82. – P.1658-1662.
[38] Davis V.L., Chan C.C., Schoen T.J., Couse J.F., Chader G.J., Korach K.S. An estrogen receptor repressor induces cataract formation in transgenic mice // *Proc. Natl. Acad. Sci. USA.* – 2002. – V.99. – N.14. – P.9427-9432.
[39] De Iongh R.U., Wederell E., Lovicu F.J., McAvoy J.W. Transforming growth factor-beta-induced epithelial-mesenchymal transition in the lens: a model for cataract formation // *Cells. Tissues. Organs.* – 2005. – V.179. – N.1-2. – P.43-55.
[40] Demir A.Y., Groothuis P.G., Nap A.W., Punyadeera C., de Goeij A.F., Evers J.L., Dunselman G.A. Menstrual effluent induces epithelial-mesenchymal transitions in mesothelial cells // *Hum. Reprod.* – 2004. – V.19. – N.1. – P.21-29.
[41] Devojno L.V., Iljuchenko R.U. *Monoaminergic systems in regulation of immune reaction.* – Novosibirsk: the Science, Siberian post, 1983.–120p.
[42] Diagnostics and treatment of internal illnesses / Edited by Komarov F.I., Gembitskogo E.V. – M.: Medicine, 1999. – V.2. – 511p.
[43] Dindjaev S.V., Pogorelov U.V. Organ complex bioamine maintenance of ovary: its components and their cooperations//*Successes of physiology sciences.* – 1993. – V.24. – N.4. – P.71-88.
[44] Donma O., Yorulmaz E., Pekel H., Suyugul N. Blood and lens lipid peroxidation and antioxidant status in normal individuals, senile and diabetic cataractous patients//*Curr. Eye Res.*–2002.–V.25.–N.1.–P.9-16.
[45] Duncan G., Collison D.J. Role of the non-neuronal cholinergic system in the eye: a review // *Life Sci.* – 2003. – V.72. – N.18-19. – P.2013-2009.
[46] Duncan G., Riach R.A., Williams M.R., Webb S.F., Dawson A.P., Reddan J.R. Calcium mobilization modulates growth of lens cells//*Cell Calcium* – 1996. – V.19. – N.1. – P.83-89.
[47] Egorova E.V., Strusova N.A., Chabrova L.S. et al. Surgical aspects of topography of anterior lens capsule // *Ophthalmology bulletin.* – 1985. – N.5. – P.11-15.
[48] Eguiagaray J.G., Egea J., Bravo-Cordero J.J., Garcia A.G. Neurotransmitters, calcium signaling and neuronal communication // *Neurocirugia* (Astur). – 2004. – V.15. – N.2. – P.109-118.

[49] Emery J. Method of preventing secondary cataracts // *Materials of conference with participation of foreign experts*: Одесса, 1987. – С.225-226.
[50] Eye diseases // Edited by T.I. Eroshevskij and A.A. Bochkareva. – *M.: Medicine*, 1977. – 264p.
[51] Fagerholm P.P., Philipson B.T. Human traumatic cataract. A quantitative microradiographic and electron microscopic study // *Acta Ophthal. (Kbh.).* – 1979. – V.57. – N.1. – P.20-32.
[52] Falk B. Observations on the possibilities of the cellular localization of monoamines by a fluorescence method // *Acta Physiol. Scand.* – 1962. – V.56. – P.197-201.
[53] Falk B., Hillarp N.A., Thieme G., Torp A. Fluorescence of catechol-amines and related compounds condensed with formaldehyde // *J. Histochem. Cytochem.* – 1962. – V.10. – P.348-354.
[54] Fedorov S.N., Panasjuk A.F., Larionov E.V. et al. Intraocular transport of substances in a pair eye // *Ophtalmosurgery.* – 1990. – N.1. – P.53-55.
[55] Formazjuk V.E. Ionic homeostasis at experimental cataract//*Materials of conference with participation of foreign experts*: Odessa, 1987. – P.42.
[56] Freel C.D., Gilliland K.O., Mekeel H.E., Giblin F.J., Costello M.J. Ultrastructural characterization and fourier analysis of fiber cell cytoplasm in the hyperbaric oxygen treated guinea pig lens opacification model // *Exp. Eye Res.* – 2003. –V.76. –N.4. – P.405-415.
[57] Freel C.D., Gilliland K.O., Wesiey Lane C., Giblin F.J., Joseph Costello M. Fourier analysis of cytoplasmic texture in nuclear fiber cells from transparent and cataractous human and animal lenses // *Exp. Eye Res.* – 2002. – V.74. –N.6. – P.689-702.
[58] Fu L., Liang J.J. Alteration of protein-protein interactions of congenital cataract crystallin mutants // *Invest. Ophthalmol. Vis. Sci.* – 2003. – V.44. – N.3. – P.1155-1159.
[59] Garus U.I. About physical inability and rehabilitation at lens diseases // *Ophtalmology J.* – 1976. – N.7. – P.530-532.
[60] Gearge A., Schmid K.L., Pow D.V. Retinal serotonin, eye growth and myopia development in chick // *Exp. Eye Res.* – 2005. – V.81. – N.5. – P.616-625.
[61] Gilliland K.O., Freel C.D., Johnsen S., Craig Fowler W., Costello M.J. Distribution, spherical structure and predicted Mie scattering of multilamellar bodies in human age-related nuclear cataracts // *Exp. Eye Res.* – 2004. – V.79. – N.4. – P.563-576.

[62] Gilliland K.O., Freel C.D., Lane C.W., Fowler W.C., Costello M.J. Multilamellar bodies as potential scattering particles in human age-related nuclear cataracts // Mol. Vis. – 2001. – V.22. – N.7. – P.120-130.
[63] Giuffre I., Taverniti L., Di Staso S. The effects of 2% ibopamine eye drops on the intraocular pressure and pupil motility of patients with open-angle glaucoma // Eur. J. Ophthalmol. – 2004. – V.14. – N.6. – P.508-513.
[64] Gordon D.S., Golubeva N.N., Sergeeva V.E. Histochemical criteria of estimation of neuromediate status in lymph organs at antigene and nonspecific influence on organism // Regulation of immune homeostasis. – L., 1982. – P.12-13.
[65] Gordon D.S., Golubeva V.F., Golubeva N.N., Sergeeva V.E. Early changes in metabolism of lymphocytes and localization adrenomediators in lymph organs at antigene influence // Early displays of fabric incompatibility. – M., 1976. – P.141-142.
[66] Gordon D.S., Sergeeva V.E. Reaction of adrenergic nervous device of thymus and spleen first minutes and hours after antigene influence // Morphological reactions of peripheral and some central departments of nervous system in norm, experiment and at various pathological processes. – Ivanovo, 1977. – P.41-43.
[67] Gordon D.S., Sergeeva V.E., Sisoiva L.A. Neuromediatore maintenance of lymph organs in norm and at antigene influence // Physiology and biochemistry in mediatore processes. – M, 1985. – 86p.
[68] Gordon D.S., Sergeeva V.E., Zelenova I.G. Neuromediators of lymph organs. – M: Science, 1982. – 128p.
[69] Goswami S., Sheets N.L., Zavadil J., Chauhan B.K., Bottinger E.P., Reddy V.N., Kantorow M., Cvekl A. Spectrum and range of oxidative stress responses of human lens epithelial cells to H2O2 insult // Jnvest. Ophthalmol. Vis. Sci. – 2003. – V.44. – N.5. – P.2084-2093.
[70] Gubler E.V., Genkin A.A. Application of criteria of nonparametric statistics for estimation of distinctions of two groups of supervision in medicobiological researches. – M, 1973. – P.3-100.
[71] Gunin A.G., Gordon D.S. Accessory of granular bioamine cells in endometrium of rats to system mononuclear phagocytes // Archive of anatomy, histology and embryology. – 1990. – V.98. – N.1. – P.68-70.
[72] Gupta P.D., Johar K. Sr., Nagpal K., Vasavada A.R. Sex hormone receptors in the human eye // Surv. Ophthalmol. – 2005. – V.50. – N.3. – P.274-284.

[73] Gupta P.D., Kalariya N., Nagpal K., Vasavada A. Pinteraction of sex steroid hormones with the eye // *Cell. Mol. Biol.* (Noisy-le-grand). – 2002. – V.48. – P.379-386.
[74] Gupta V., Wagner B.J. Expression of the functional glucocorticoid receptor in mouse and human lens epithelial cells // *Jnvest. Ophthalmol. Vis. Sci.* – 2003. – V.44. – N.5. – P.2041-2046.
[75] Gushin G.V. Adrenergic and cholinergic mechanisms of regulation of functions lymph cells: *The author's abstract dissertation.* – S.-Pb., 1992. – 36p.
[76] Ham A., Kormak D. Histology // *Fundamental monography in five volumes.* – M: World, 1983. – V.5. – 294p.
[77] Hanna C., O´Brien J.E. Cell production and migration in the epithelial layer of the lens // *Arch. Ophthal.* – 1961. – V.66. –N.1. – P.129-133.
[78] Happe V. Ophtalmology // *Directory of the practical doctor.* – M: Medical Press-Inform, 2005. – 352p.
[79] Hasko G., Elenkou I.J., Vizi E.S. Presynaptic receptors involved in the modulation of release of noradrenaline from the sympathetic nerve terminals of the rat thymus // *Immunol. Lett.* – 1995. – V.47. – N.1-2. – P.33-137.
[80] Haus C., Galand A. Mitomycin against posterior capsular opacification: an experimental study in rabbits // *Brit. J. Ophthal.* – 1996. – V.80. – N.12. – P.1087-1091.
[81] Hayashi H., Hayashi K., Nakao F. et al. Quantitative comparison of posterior capsule opacification after polymethilmethacrylate, silicone and soft acryl intraocular lens implantation // *Arch. Ophthal.* – 1998. – V.116. – N.12. – P.1579-1582.
[82] Humphry R., Ball S., Brammal J. et al. Lens epithelial cells adhere less to HEMA then to PMMA intraocular lenses//*Eye.* – 1995.–V.5. – N.1. – P.66-69.
[83] Ibaraki N., Li-Ren L., Reddy V. Effect of growth factors on proliferation and differentiation in human lens epithelial cells in early subculture // *Invest. Ophthal. Vis. Sci.* – 1995. – V.36. – P.2304-2312.
[84] Ibaraki N., Ohara K., Miyamoto T. Membranous outgrowth suggesting lens epithelial cells proliferation in pseudophakic eyes // *Amer. J. Ophthal.* – 1995. – V.119. – N.6. – P.706-711.
[85] Jurina N.A., Radostina A.I. Connecting tissue. *Development, structure and functions of cells and intercellular substance:* Manual. – M: Publishing House of People's Friendship University of Russia, 1987. – 54p.

[86] Jurina N.A., Radostina A.I. *Mast cells and their role in an organism.* – M, 1977. – 238p.
[87] Jurina N.A., Radostina A.I. Participation of mast cells in reactions to antigene and stressful influences // *Physiology of immune homeostasis.* – Rostov on Don. – 1977. – P.88-89.
[88] Kaisho Y., Watanabe T., Nakata M., Yano T., Yasuhara Y., Shimakawa K., Mori I., Sakura Y., Terao Y., Matsui H., Taketomi S. Transgenic rats overexpressing the human MrgX3 gene show cataracts and abnormal skin phenotype // *Biochem. Biophys. Res. Commun.* – 2005. – V.330. – N.3. – P.653-657.
[89] Kalinin A.P., Mozherenkov V.P., Prokophfieva G.L. Eyes – the card of endocrine diseases. – M: *Medical newspaper*, 1995. – 61p.
[90] Karnaukhov V.N. Luminescent spectral analysis of cell. – M.: *Science*, 1978. – 208p.
[91] Kashintseva L.T., Teljushenko V.D. Features of condition trophism of anterior chamber and lens at patients with ecsfolyative glaucoma // *Ophtalmology J.* – 1999. – N.6. – P.363-368.
[92] Kato K., Kurosaka D., Nagamoto T. Apoptotic cell death in rabbit lens after lens extraction//*Invest. Ophthal. Vis. Sci.*–1997. – V.38.–N.11. – P. 2322-2330.
[93] Khamidova M.H. *Development of eye and optic-conduction ways at the person.* – Tashkent: Medicine, 1972. – 73p.
[94] Kogan M.Z. Biological meaning of histamine // *Lab. Thing.* – 1987. – N.9. – P.712-714.
[95] Koreneva E.A., Shekojan V.A. Regulation of protective functions in organism. – L.: *Science*, 1982. – 139p.
[96] Korsakova N.V. Morphofunctional characteristic a histamine-containing structures of lens in early terms of chemical irritation in eye // *Morphology.* – S.-Pb.: Esculap, 2004. – V.126. – N.6. – P.37-39.
[97] Korsakova N.V., Sergeeva V.E. Histamine-containing structures of lens in intact rats // *Morphology.* – S.-Pb.: Esculap, 2004. – V.125. – N.5. – P.27-30.
[98] Kovalev I.F. Pathogenesis of beam cataracts: *The author's abstract dissertation.* – Odessa, 1967. – 37p.
[99] Kovalev I.F. *Functional mechanisms development of radio-biological effects.* – M: Atomedit, 1969. – 310p.
[100] Kurisheva N.I. Pseudoecsfoliative syndrome//*Bulletin of ophthalmology.* – 2001. – N.3. – P.47-50.

[101] Kurisheva N.I., Fedorov A.A., Erichev V.P. Pathomorphologic features of anterior and posterior capsule of cataract lens at with primary glaucoma // *Glaucoma. Material Russia conf.*, M. – 1999. – P.263-266.
[102] Kurisheva N.I., Fedorov A.A., Erichev V.P. Pathomorphologic aspects of cataract lens at glaucoma//*Ophthalmology bulletin.* – 2000. – V.116. – N.2. – P.13-16.
[103] Kurosaka D., Kato K., Nagamoto T., Negishi K. Growth factors influence contractility and α-smooth muscle actin expression in bovine lens epithelial cells // *Invest. Ophthal. Vis. Sci.* – 1995. – V.36. – N.8. – P.1701-1708.
[104] Kurosaka D., Kato K., Nagamoto T. Presence of α-smooth muscle actin in lens epithelial cells of aphakic rabbit eyes//*Brit. J. Ophthal.* – 1996. – V.80. – N.10. – P.906-910.
[105] Kvetnaja T.V., Knjazkin I.V., Kvetnoj I.M. Melatonine – *Neuroimmunoendocryne marker of an age pathology.* – S.-Pb.: Publishing House DEAN, 2005. – 144p.
[106] Larionov E.V., Panasjuk A.F., Tumanjan V. et al. The Experimental secondary cataract induced by immune complexes // *Bulletin of ophthalmology.* – 1989. – N.6. – P.53-56.
[107] Lebehov P.I., Kugleev A.A, Vladimirova L.V., Fajnshtejn E.J. About aftersurgery treatment at cataract // *Bulletin of ophthalmology.* – 1983. – N.4. – P.71.
[108] Lee S.M., Tseng L.M., Li A.F., Liu H.C., Liu T.Y., Chi C.W. Polymorphism of estrogen metabolism genes and cataract // *Med. Hypotheses.* – 2004. – V.63. – N.3. – P.494-497.
[109] Libman E.S., Shahova E.V. Status and dynamics of blindness and invalidity owing to organ of vision pathology in Russia // *VII Congress ophtalmol. In Russia: Theses of reports.* – 2000. – Part 2. – P.209-214.
[110] Linnik L.F., Ostrovsky M.A. et al. IOL absorbing ultra-violet beams: safety, efficiency and use prospect in ophtalmosurgery (the literature review) // *Ophthalmosurgery:* M, 1991. – N.4. – P.3-7.
[111] Lipschitz D.L., Crowley W.R., Bealer S.L. Differential sensitivity of intranuclear and systemic oxytocin release to central noradrenergic receptor stimulation durig mid- and late gestation in rats // *Am. J. Physiol. Endjcrinol. Metab.* – 2004. – V.287. – N.3. – P.523-528.
[112] Lopashov G.V, Stroev O.G. *Growth of eye in the experimental researches.* – M: Publishing House AN of the USSR, 1963. – 205p.

[113] Lorand L., Conrad S.M., Velasco P.T. Formation of a 55,000-weight cross-linked beta-crystallin dimer in the Ca2+-treated lens. A model for cataract // *Biochemistry.* – 1985. – V.24. – V.6. – P.1525-1531.
[114] Lorand L., Conrad S.M., Velasco P.T. Inhibition of beta-crystallin cross-linking in the Ca2+-treated lens // *Invest. Ophthalmol. Vis. Sci.* – 1987. – V.28. – N.7. – P.1218-1222.
[115] Lovicu F., Chamberlain C., McAvoy J. Differential effects of aqueous and vitreous on fiber differentiation and extracellular matrix accumulation in lens epithelial explants // *Invest. Ophthal. Vis. Sci.* – 1995. – V.36. – N.7. – P.1459-1469.
[116] Lovicu F., McAvoy J. Growth factor regulation of lens development // *Dev. Biol.* – 2005. – V.280. – N.1. – P.1-14.
[117] Lubovtseva L.A. *Luminescent-histochemical research amines-containing structures of marrow, thymus and blood at action neuromediators and antigenes.* – Cheboksary: Publishing House the Chuvash Stat Un-ty, 1993. – 100p.
[118] Lui P.P., Chan F.L., Suen Y.K., Kwok T.T., Kong S.K. The nucleus of HeLa cells contains tubular structures for Ca2+-signaling with the involvement of mitochondria // *Biochem. Biophys. Res. Commun.* – 2003. – V.308. – N.4. – P.826-833.
[119] Maltsev E.V., Pavljuchenko K.P. *Biological features and diseases of lens.* – Odessa: Astroprint, 2002. – 448p.
[120] Marchini G., Babighian S., Tosi R., Perfetti S., Bonomi L. Comparative study of the effects of 2% ibopamine, 10% phenylephrine, and 1% tropicamide on the anterior segment // *Invest. Ophthalmol. Vis. Sci.* – 2003. – V.44. – N.1. – P.281-289.
[121] Matsuura H., Matsuto T. Electron microscopic studies on the epithelial cells of human cataract//*Acta Soc. Ophthal. Jap.* – 1975. – V.79. – N.9. – P.1340-1343.
[122] Maychuk J.F. Preventive of blindness as a problem of international healthcare // *Bulletin of ophthalmology.* – 1980. – N.3. – P.59-62.
[123] McAvoy J.W. The spatial relationships between presumptive lens and optic vesicle/cup during early eye morphogenesis in the rat // *Exp. Eye Res.* – 1981. –V.33. – N.4. – P.447-458.
[124] McAvoy J.W., Chamberlain C., Richardson M.A., Lovicu F.J. Fibroblast growth factor (FGF): a lens-inducing molecule from the retina. // *Excerpta medica:* Amsterdam, 1991. – P.627-631.
[125] Mejerson F.Z. *Adaptation, stress and prophylaxis.* – M: Science, 1981. – 277p.

[126] Mirshahi M., Agarwal M.K. Receptor-mediated adrenocorticoid hormone signaling in ocular tissues // *Biochem. Pharmacol.* – 2003. – V.65. – N.8. – P.1207-1214.
[127] Miyano K., Chiou G.C. Pharmacological prevention of ocular inflammation induced by lens proteins // *Ophthalmic. Res.* – 1984. – V.16. – N.5. – P.256-263.
[128] Nielsen H.L., Gudjonsson T., Villadsen R., Ronnov-Jessen L., Petersen O.W. Collagen gel contraction serves to rapidly distinguish epithelial- and mesenchymal-derived cells irrespective of α-smooth muscle actin expression // *In Vitro Cell Dev. Biol. Anim.* – 2003. – V.39. – N.7. – P.297-303.
[129] Nishi O., Nishi K., Fujiwara T., Shirosava E. Types of collagen synthesized by the lens epithelial cells of human cataract // *Brit. J. Ophthal.* – 1995. – V.79. – N.10. – P.939-943.
[130] Nishi O., Nishi K., Fujiwara T. et al. Effects of the cytokines on the proliferation of and collagen synthesis by human cataract lens epithelial cells // *Brit. J. Ophthal.* – 1996. – V.80. – N.1. – P.63-68.
[131] Nishi O., Nishi K., Imanishi M. et al. Effect of cytokines on the prostagland in E2 synthesis by lens epithelial cells of human cataract // *Brit. J. Ophthal.* – 1995. – V.79. – N. 10. – P.934-938.
[132] Nowak J., Nawrocki J. Histamine in the human eye // *Ophthalmic. Res.* – 1987. – V.19. – N.2. – P.72-75.
[133] Ogueta S.B., Schwartz S.D., Yamashita C.K., Farber D.B. Estrogen receptor in the human eye: influence of gender and age on gene expression // *Invest. Ophthalmol. Vis. Sci.* – 1999. – V.40. – N.9. – P.1906-1911.
[134] Ohata H., Tanaka K., Aizawa H., Ao Y., Iijima T., Momose K. Lysophosphatidic acid sensitises Ca2+ influx through mechanosensitive ion channels in cultured lens epithelial cells // *Cell. Signal.* – 1997. – V.9. – N.8. – P.609-616.
[135] Petrovich J.A., Borovik G.A. Enzymes of carbohydrate exchange and ATF in eye at infringement of its innervation//*Reports of AS the USSR.* – M, 1973. – V.212. – N.6. – P.1465-1468.
[136] Pirie A., R. van Heyningen. *Eye biochemistry.* – M: Medicine, 1968. – 400p.
[137] Polunin G.S, Ivanov M.N. About lekozim influence on a lens // *Bulletin of ophthalmology.* – 1986. – V.102. – N.6. – P.42-44.

[138] Polunin G.S, Nurieva O.M. Capabilities of lekozim for conservative treatment of senile cataract // *Materials of conf. by foreign specialists: Theses of reports.* – Odessa, 1987. – P.52-53.
[139] Polunin G.S. About lekozom influence on a current of some kinds of cataracts//*Bulletin of ophthalmology.* – 1989. – V.105. – N.4. – P.44-48.
[140] Preston Mason R., Tulenko T.N., Jacob R.F. Direct evidence for cholesterol crystalline domains in biologic membranes: role in human pathobiology // *Biochim. Biophys. Acta.* – 2003. – V.1610. – N.2. – P.198-207.
[141] Puchkovskaja N.A. Cataract – the basic removable reason of blindness // *Ophthalmology J.* – 1983. – N.8. – P.449-452.
[142] Puchkovskaja N.A., Krasnovid T.A., Usov N.I., Kravchenko Л.И. About the regularity developments of age cataracts // *Materials of VII congress of ophthalmology in Ukraine*: Odessa. – 1990. – P.262-263.
[143] Qu B., Zhang J.S. Expression and role of inositol 1,4,5-trisphosphate receptor and ryanodine receptor in a human lens epithelial cell line // *Zhonghua. Yan. Ke. Za. Zhi.* – 2003. – V.39. – N.7. – P.389-394.
[144] Rabinovich M.G. *Cataract.* – M: Medicine, 1965. – 172p.
[145] Rapis E.G., Tumanov V.P., Levin J.M., Kurbanov N.H. Management lymphatic of eye with help of dalargin // *Bulletin of experimental biology and medicine.* – 1990. – V.110. – N.10. – P.436-438.
[146] Riach R.A., Duncan G., Williams M.R., Webb S.F. Histamine and ATP mobilize calcium by activation of H1 and P2U receptors in human lens epithelial cells // *J. Physiol.* – 1995. – V.486. – N.2. – P.273-282.
[147] Richardson N., McAvoy J. Age-related changes in fibre differentiation of rat lens epithelial cells in vitro // *Exp. Eye Res.* – 1988. – V.46. – P.259-267.
[148] Richardson N., McAvoy J. Age-related changes in fibre differentiation of rat lens epithelial explants exposed to fibroblast growth factor // *Exp. Eye Res.* – 1990. – V.50. – N.2. – P.203-211.
[149] Romase B. *Microscopic technics.* – M: Publishing House of the foreign literature. 1954.
[150] Ronkina T.I., Chabrova L.S., Borisova L.M. Biomechanical properties of lens capsule at emmetropia and myopia//*Ophthalmologic J.* – 1989. – N.7. – P.420-425.
[151] Ronkina T.I., Vasin V.I, Karoev O.A. Features of ultrastructure of posterior capsule of lens in age aspect and at various kinds of cataracts // *Ophthalmologic J.* – 1985. – N.6. – P.358-361.

[152] Rujoi M., Jin J., Borchman D., Tang D., Yappert M.C. Isolation and lipid characterization of cholesterol-enriched fractions in cortical and nuclear human lens fibers//*Invest. Ophthalmol. Vis. Sci.*–2003. – V.44. – N.4. – P.1634-1642.
[153] Saika S., Kono-Saika S., Ohnishi Y., Sato M., Muragaki Y., Ooshima A., Flanders K.C., Yoo J., Anzano M., Liu C.Y., Kao W.W., Roberts A.B. Smad3-signaling is required for epithelial-mesenchymal transition of lens epithelium after injury // *Am. J. Pathol.* – 2004. – V.164. – N.2. – P.651-663.
[154] Saika S., Miyamoto T., Tanaka S., Tanaka T., Ishida I., Ohnishi Y., Ooshima A., Ishiwata T., Asano G., Chikama T., Shiraishi A., Liu C.Y., Kao C.W., Kao W.W. Response of lens epithelial cells to injury: role of lumican in epithelial mesenchymal transition // *Invest. Ophthalmol. Vis. Sci.* – 2003. – V.44. – N.5. – P.2094-2102.
[155] Saika S., Tanaka S., Miyamoto T. et al. Lens epithelial cell proliferation and extracellular matrix accumulation on intra ocular lenses and residual lens capsules in humans // *In: XI-th Congress of the European Society of Ophthalmology.* – Budapest, 1997. – N.1112. – P.341.
[156] Sakaue T., Ohhira M., Ogata K., Ohmori S. Physiological activities of S-(1,2-dicarboxyethyl)glutathione as an intrinsic tripeptide present in liver, heart and lens // *Arzneimittelforschung.* – 1992. – V.42. – N.12. – P.1482-1486.
[157] Samadi A., Cenedella R.J., Carlson C.G. Diethylstilbestrol increases intracellular calcium in lens epithelial cells // *Pflugers Arch.* – 2005. – V.450. – N.3. – P.145-154.
[158] Schein O., West S., Munoz B. et al. Cortical lenticular opacification distribution and location in a longitudinal study // *Invest. Ophthal. Vis. Sci.* – 1994. – V.35. – N.2. – P.363-366.
[159] Schlotzer-Schrechardt U.M., Mark K. von., Sakai L., Naumann J. Increased extracellular deposition of fibrilline-containing fibrils in pseudoexfoliation syndrome//*Invest. Ophthal. Vis. Sci.* – 1997. – V.38. – N.5. – P.970-984.
[160] Selgas R., Bajo M.A., Aguilera A., Sanchez-Tomero J.A., Cirugeda A., del Peso G., Alvarez V., Jimenez-Heffernan J.A., Diaz C., Lopez-Cabrera M. Epithelial-mesenchymal transition in fibrosing processes. Mesothelial cells obtained ex vivo from patients treated with peritoneal dialysis as transdifferentiation model // *Nefrologia.* – 2004. – V.24. – N.1. – P.34-39.

[161] Sergeeva V.E, Mihajlova I.M., Timofeeva G.M. Getting together the monoamines in parenchyma of thyroid on lipide-containing complex connections // Makro- and microstructure of tissues in norm, pathology and experiment/*Chuvash Stat University.*–Cheboksary, 1975. – P.71-78.
[162] Sergeeva V.E, Gordon D.S., Sysoeva L.A., Gordon B.M. Reaction of a bioamines-containing structures lymphadens at first hour of contact of organism with an antigene // *Reports of scientific conference "Gistogenez and regeneration."* – L, 1986. – P.23-24.
[163] Sergeeva V.E, Gordon D.S., Vozjakova T.R., Gordon B.M. Reaction of structural bioamines and prostaglandin E2 of thymus on antigene stimulus // *Reports of the Russia congress of anatomists, histologists and embriologists.* – L., 1988. – P.112.
[164] Sergeeva V.E, Sysoyev L.A. Monoaminy of thymus and spleen in early terms after heart allotransplantation // *Early displays of tissue incompatibility.* – M, 1979. – P.83-84.
[165] Sergeeva V.E, Vozjakova T.R. Luminescent-histochemical research of rat's thymus after introduction of soluble gamma globulin // *Morphology of compensation processes* / Ivanovo medical institute.–Ivanovo, 1987. – P.90-92.
[166] Sergeeva V.E, Vozjakova T.R. Luminiscent-histochemical analysis of bioamines in structures of thymus at 15 minutes after introduction of a soluble antigene // *Luminescent analysis in medicine, biology and its hardware maintenance.* – Riga: RMI, 1985. – P.119-120.
[167] Sergeeva V.E, Vozjakova T.R., Sergeeva A.T. Functional communication of thymus and lymphaden on maintenance neuromediators // *Phisiology and biochemistry of mediate processes.* – M, 1990. – P.264-265.
[168] Sergeeva V.E. Luminescent morphology and adrenergic innervation of thymus: *The dissertation Author's abstract.* – M, 1976. – 20p.
[169] Sergeeva V.E. The quantitative and qualitative analysis monoamines of adrenergic structures of thymus // *Macro- and microstructure of tissues in norm, pathology and experiment* / Chuvash Stait University. – Cheboksary, 1979. – P.11-14.
[170] Shearer T., Anderson R. Histologic changes during senile cataractogenesis: A light microscopy study // *Exp. Eye Res.* – 1985. – V.40. – P.557-565.
[171] Shiljaev R.R., Vinogradov S.J., Vinogradova E.E. Neuromediatorical bioamines and their value in diagnostics of children diseases // *Bulletin of the Ivanovo medical academy.* – 1996. – V.1. – N.2. – P.81-88.

[172] Shlenskaya O.V., Pozdeeva N.A. Estimation of hemato-ophthalmic barrier at age macular dystrophies according to laser tyndallimetria // *Questions of clinical and experimental medicine: Materials of regional scientifically-practical conference.* – Cheboksary: Publishing House of the Chuvash State University, 2009. – P.173-176.

[173] Shvalev V.N. Some morphological bases of the doctrine about trophic function of nervous system // *Archive of anatomy, histology, embryology.* – M, 1971. – N.8. – P.8-29.

[174] Smallhorn M., Murray M.J., Saint R. The epithelial-mesenchymal transition of the drosophila mesoderm requires the Rho GTP exchange factor Pebble // *Development.* – 2004. – V.131. – N.11. – P.2641-2651.

[175] Smorodchenko A.T. Lymph node in norm and at antigene influences // *The Manual* / Chuvash Stat University. – Cheboksary, 1996. – 76p.

[176] Solomonova V.G, Sorokin L.V. Interaction of mediatorical systems, a hypothesis, the facts // *Physiology and biochemistry of mediatorical processes: Theses of the report of 5th All-Union conference.*–M, 1990. – P.281.

[177] Somov E.E. *Clinical's anatomy of an organ of vision of the person.* – M: MEDICAL PRESS-INFORM, 2005. – 136p.

[178] Spassky A.S. Technique of estimation of irritating action of chemical substances on anterior department of eye//*Hygiene and sanitary.*–1992. – N.3. – P.75-77.

[179] Stone R.A., Sugimoto R., Gill A.S., Liu J., Capehart C., Lindstrom J.M. Effects of nicotinic antagonists on ocular growth and experimental myopia//*Invest. Ophthalmol. Vis. Sci.*–*2001.*–V.42. – N.3. – P.557-565.

[180] Stuck H., Hammer U. Einfluss des diabetes mellitus auf das vordere zentrale Linsenepithel bei Katarakt patienten//*Der Ophthalmologe.* – 1997. – Bd.94. – N.5. – S.327-331.

[181] Stukalov S.E., Sudovskaya T.V. Immunological aspects pathogenesis and treatments exudative reactions at implantation intraocular lenses // *Bulletin of ophthalmology.* – 1993. – V.109. – N.3. – P.12-14.

[182] Suslikov V.L., Andreev A.N., Stepanov R.V. et al. To a question on a role of biogeochemical factors in pathogenesis of an age cataract // *Ophthalmologic J.* – 1990. – N.5. – P.296-299.

[183] Synder A., Omulecka A., Ratynska M., Omulecki W. A study of human lens epithelial cells by light and electron microscopy and by immunohistochemistry in different types of cataracts//*Klin. Oczna.* – 2002. – V.104. – N.5-6. – P.369-373.

[184] Takamura Y., Sugimoto Y., Kubo E., Takahashi Y., Akagi Y. Immunohistochemical study of apoptosis of lens epithelial cells in human and diabetic rat cataracts//*Nippon. Ganka. Gakkai. Zasshi.*–2000. – V.104. – N.4. – P.221-225.
[185] Thiery J.P. Epithelial-mesenchymal transitions in development and pathologies//*Curr. Opin. Cell. Biol.* – 2003. – V.15. – N.6. – P.740-746.
[186] Tokin I.B. Electric-microscope analysis of process of cells differentiation and dedifferentiation // *Archive of anatomy, histology, embryology.* – M, 1972. – N.6. – P.46-62.
[187] Udenfriend S. *Fluorescent analysis in biology and medicine.* – M: World, 1965. – 484p.
[188] Uga S., Tsuchiya K., Ishikawa S. Histopathological study of Emory mouse cataract//*Albrecht V. Graefes Arch. Klin. Exp. Ophthal.* – 1988. – Bd.226. – S.15-27.
[189] Unakar N., Harries W., Tsui J. Acid phosphatase. II. Cytochemical localization in lenses of normal and galactose-fed rats//*Exp. Eye Res.* – 1985. – V.40. – N.1. – P.117-126.
[190] Venkataswamy G., Lepkowski J., Rawilla T. et al. Rapid epidemiological assessment of cataract blindness//*Intern. J. Epidemiol.*–1989. – V.18. – N.4. – P.661-667.
[191] Vinogradov S.U., Pogorelov U.V. Serotonine and its participation in functional regulation of thyroid gland // *Success of modern biology.* – 1984. – V.98. – N.2. – P.206-218.
[192] Vinogradov S.U., Pogorelov U.V., Torshilova I.U. Functional morphology neuromediate bioamine maintenance of thyroid gland during the pregnancy // *Bulletin of the Ivanovo medical academy.* – 1996. – V.7. – N.1. – P.23-27.
[193] Vojno-Jaseneckij V.V. *Growth and variability of eye's fabrics at its diseases and traumas.* – Kiev: Visha School, 1979. – 224p.
[194] Volkova O.V. *Neurodistrophic process.* – M.: Medicine, 1978. – p.256.
[195] Wang L., Wormstone I.M., Reddan J.R., Duncan G. Growth factor receptor signaling in human lens cells: role of the calcium store // *Exp. Eye Res.* – 2005. – V.80. – N.6. – P.885-895.
[196] Wang X., Simpkins J.W., Dykens J.A., Cammarata P.R. Oxidative damage to human lens epithelial cells in culture: estrogen protection of mitochondrial potential, ATP, and cell viability // *Invest. Ophthalmol. Vis. Sci.* – 2003. – V.44. – N.5. – P.2067-2075.
[197] Weale R. Senescent vision: is it all the fault of the lens // *Eye.* – 1987. – N.1. – P.217-221.

[198] Wiekham L.A., Gao J., Toda I., Rocha E.M., Ono M., Sullivan D.A. Identification of androgen, estrogen and progesterone receptor mRNAs in the eye//*Acta. Ophthalmol. Scand.*–2000. – V.78. – N.2. – P.146-153.

[199] Willekens B., Vrensen G. The origin of Elschnig pearls//*Ophthal. Res.* – 1999. – N.156. – P.29.

[200] Williams M.R., Riach R.A., Collison D.J., Duncan G. Role of the endoplasmic reticulum in shaping calcium dynamics in human lens cells // *Invest. Ophthalmol. Vis. Sci.* – 2001. – V.42. – N.5. – P.1009-1017.

[201] Wisfeld I.L., Kassile G.N. *Histamine in biochemistry and physiology.* – M.: Science, 1981. - 227p.

[202] Yamamoto K., Shinosaki K., Hori S., Kobayashi M. Apoptosis in lens epithelial cell obtained during cataract surgery // *Congr. Europ. Soc. Ophthal. XIII-th: Final program an abstract book.* – Istanbul, 2001. – P.224.

[203] Yildirim N., Ozer A., Inal M., Angin K., Yurdakul S. The effect of N-acetyl serotonin on ultraviolet-radiation-induced cataracts in rats // *Ophthalmologica.* – 2003. – V.217. – N.2. – P.148-153.

[204] Zhang X.H., Sun H.M., Ji J., Zhang H., Ma W.J., Jin Z., Yuan J.Q. Sex hormones and their receptors in patients with age-related cataract // *J. Cataract. Refract. Surg.* – 2003. – V.29. – N.1. – P.71-77.

[205] Zhuravleva Z.N. Ultrastructure of synapses in the transplants of nervous tissue, developing in anterior chamber of eye // *Ontohenesis.* – 1987. – V.18. – N.6. – P.631-638.

Index

A

accommodation, 9, 10
acetaldehyde, 61
acetylcholine, 22, 25, 60
acid, 11, 69
activity level, 22
adaptation, xiii
adenosine, 11
adrenaline, 23
Africa, xi
age, vii, ix, xi, xii, xiii, 5, 7, 9, 10, 14, 15, 16, 17, 18, 23, 24, 27, 28, 31-36, 40-45, 47, 51, 52, 53, 59, 61, 63, 64, 67, 69, 70, 73, 75
aggregation, 14, 18
amine(s), vii, xii, 6, 21, 22, 24, 32, 42, 68
amino, 29
amphibia, 60
anatomy, 60, 64, 73, 74
androgen, 75
androgenic, xii, 11, 42
antigen, 29
antioxidant, 14, 24, 62
apoptosis, 3, 6, 74
aqueous humor, 10, 12
assessment, 74
ATF, 69
atmosphere, 17
ATP, 11, 13, 18, 43, 70, 74

B

base, 29
beams, 67
biochemistry, 39, 64, 69, 72, 73, 75
biosynthesis, 24
birds, 4
blindness, xi, 67, 68, 70, 74
blood, 2, 24, 42, 68
brain, 59
browsing, 33, 34
bursa, 2

C

Ca^{2+}, 61, 68, 69
calcium, xii, 12, 13, 14, 22, 23, 39, 41, 42, 43, 61, 62, 70, 74, 75
calcium channel blocker, 13
capsule, xii, 2, 3, 4, 6, 9, 10, 13, 14, 15, 16, 18, 19, 20, 24, 31, 40, 41, 50, 51, 53, 62, 65, 67, 70
carbohydrate, 69
cataract extraction, 7
catecholamines, 28, 33, 34, 35, 42, 43, 47, 53, 63
cell death, 66, 70
central nervous system, 21
chemical(s), 4, 6, 12, 23, 60, 61, 66, 73

chemicals, 60
cholesterol, 13, 14, 15, 70, 71
circadian rhythm(s), 21, 24
clusters, 3
collagen, 6, 10, 15, 18, 19, 20, 69
color, 16, 17, 28, 33, 40
communication, 62, 72
compensation, 72
complications, xi, 6, 19, 61
compounds, 63
compression, 32
condensation, 28
conductance, 59
conduction, 66
conference, 61, 63, 72, 73
congenital cataract, 63
congress, 61, 70, 71, 72
control group, 27
cornea, 9, 17, 27
correlations, 23
cortex, 4, 10, 16, 33, 40, 49, 50, 51, 52
covering, 32
crescentic glomerulonephritis, 60
crystalline, 23, 60, 70
cultivation, 5, 41
culture, 4, 20, 44, 61, 74
cytokines, 69
cytoplasm, 3, 14, 15, 16, 22, 36, 40, 41, 57, 63

D

defects, 5, 19
dehydration, 29, 31, 32
deoxyribonucleic acid (DNA), 2
depolarization, 10
deposition, 71
deposits, 15
deprivation, 25
developing countries, xi
deviation, 32
diabetes, 15, 73
diabetic cataract, 62
dialysis, 71

diseases, xiii, 11, 17, 19, 39, 44, 63, 66, 68, 72, 74
dislocation, 4
dispersion, 60
dissociation, 16, 32, 40, 51
distribution, 3, 11, 12, 60, 61, 71
DNA, 2
drainage, 12
drinking water, 17
drying, 28

E

E-cadherin, 20
ectoderm, 1, 2, 5
edema, 16
effluent, 62
electron, 63, 73
electron microscopy, 73
embryogenesis, 1, 2, 3, 5
embryology, 64, 73, 74
endocrine, xii, 24, 32, 59, 66
endocrine system, xii, 59
endothelial cells, 24
endothelium, 4
energy, 17
epithelial cells, xii, 2, 3, 4, 5, 6, 10, 11, 12, 13, 15, 20, 22, 32, 36, 41, 44, 45, 47, 50, 60, 64, 65, 67, 68, 69, 70, 71, 73, 74
epithelium, 1, 3, 4, 6, 7, 10, 11, 14, 15, 24, 25, 32, 35, 43, 49, 50, 51, 52, 53, 60, 71
estrogen, 18, 60, 62, 67, 74, 75
estrogenic, xii, 11, 12, 18, 42
ethanol, 28, 29
etiology, 25
evidence, ix, 12, 22, 23, 24, 32, 40, 41, 42, 43, 47, 70
evolution, 45
experimental condition, 59
extracellular matrix, 68, 71
extraction, 6, 19, 28, 66

Index

F

fiber(s), 2, 3, 4, 5, 9, 10, 13, 14, 15, 16, 18, 23, 32, 33, 35, 36, 39, 41, 43, 50, 51, 52, 57, 63, 68, 71
fibroblast growth factor, 70
fibroblasts, 4, 5, 15, 18, 19
fibrosis, xii, 6, 18, 19, 20
fluid, 4
fluorescence, 27, 28, 33, 35, 61, 63
fluorine, 14, 17
food, 14
formaldehyde, 28, 63
formation, vii, ix, xii, xiii, 1, 2, 3, 4, 6, 10, 11, 15, 16, 18, 19, 20, 23, 28, 31, 32, 33, 34, 35, 36, 40, 41, 43, 44, 45, 47, 61, 62
Fourier analysis, 63
fragments, 15
France, 19
free radicals, 24

G

gamma globulin, 72
gastrointestinal tract, 17
gastrulation, 20
gene expression, 59, 69
glaucoma, xi, 16, 19, 22, 23, 64, 66, 67
glomerulonephritis, 20
glutathione, 13, 71
glycerin, 29
glycogen, 15, 18, 41
glycosaminoglycans, 4
granules, 18, 36, 41
Great Britain, 29
growth, xii, 3, 4, 5, 6, 11, 12, 22, 25, 42, 50, 51, 62, 63, 65, 68, 73
growth factor, xii, 3, 4, 5, 6, 11, 12, 22, 42, 62, 65, 68

H

hemorrhage, 23
heterogeneity, 11
histamine, xii, 6, 12, 13, 21, 22, 23, 24, 27, 28, 33, 34, 35, 42, 43, 47, 53, 61, 66
histology, 64, 73, 74
homeostasis, 18, 63, 64, 66
hormone(s), xii, 18, 32, 42, 64, 65, 69, 75
House, 65, 67, 68, 70, 73
human, vii, ix, xi, xii, xiii, 2, 5, 6, 7, 9, 10, 11, 12, 13, 18, 20, 21, 22, 23, 31, 35, 36, 43, 44, 45, 47, 51, 52, 53, 60, 61, 63, 64, 65, 66, 68, 69, 70, 71, 73, 74, 75
humoral regulation, xii, 42
humoral system, xii, 21, 42
hydrogen, 29, 41
hyperglycemia, 17
hypertension, 17
hypothesis, 73

I

identification, 12, 27
immune reaction, 62
immune system, xii, 32
immunofluorescence, 12
immunohistochemistry, 73
in vitro, 24, 41, 60, 70
incompatibility, 64, 72
individuals, 62
induction, 4, 7
inductor, 4
inflammation, 69
inhibition, 13, 20, 59
injury(s), 5, 6, 11, 14, 18, 20, 24, 41, 44, 71
inositol, 70
institutions, ix
integrity, 7, 18
interference, 28
intracellular calcium, 71
intraocular, xii, 6, 12, 16, 19, 23, 24, 42, 60, 64, 65, 73
intraocular pressure, 12, 23, 24, 42, 64
inversion, 4
involution, 45
ions, xii, 12, 13, 14, 22, 23, 42
iris, 1, 5, 9, 15, 21, 50, 69
irradiation, 17

J

Japan, 18

K

K^+, 59
keratinocytes, 4

L

larvae, 6
lead, 12
learning, ix
lens opacity, xii, xiii, 15, 17, 39, 42, 45
lenticular cells, xii, 50
light, 6, 10, 17, 24, 28, 35, 62, 72, 73
lipid peroxidation, 14, 62
lipids, 14
liver, 17, 71
localization, 12, 22, 31, 36, 40, 60, 61, 63, 64, 74
longitudinal study, 71
lymph, 64, 65
lymphocytes, 64

M

macromolecules, 24
magnesium, 13, 14
magnitude, 33
mammal, 6
marrow, 68
mast cells, 66
matrix, 1, 6
measurement, 28
medical, ix, 72, 74
medicine, vii, ix, 39, 40, 43, 70, 72, 73, 74
melatonin, 24
mellitus, 15, 73
membranes, xii, 9, 10, 13, 14, 16, 22, 31, 33, 39, 43, 70
menstruation, 20

mesoderm, 73
metabolism, xiii, 12, 13, 25, 64, 67
methanol, 29
mice, 3, 59, 62
microscope, 27, 28, 74
microscopy, 6, 14, 16, 18, 22, 31, 33, 35, 41, 72
microstructure, 72
microtome, 29
migration, 65
mitochondria, 2, 11, 12, 22, 68
mitochondrial DNA, 24
mitosis, 2
models, 41
molecular biology, 4, 39
monolayer, 10
morbidity, xi, 17, 18
morphogenesis, 19, 45, 68
morphology, 4, 6, 18, 20, 40, 72, 74
mRNAs, 75
mucosa, 61
mucus, 12
multicellular organisms, 19, 20
muscarinic receptor, 61
myoblasts, 4
myofibroblasts, 6, 15, 19, 20, 44
myopia, 18, 25, 63, 70, 73

N

Na^+, 59
natural science, 39
neoplasm, 19
nerve, 65
nervous system, xii, xiii, 64, 73
neuroectodermic tissue, 4
neurons, 12, 60
neurotransmitters, 21
neutral, 28
nicotine, 25
nuclear membrane, 22
nuclei, 2, 3, 4, 12, 15, 22, 32
nucleus, 2, 3, 10, 15, 16, 22, 32, 33, 40, 50, 51, 52, 68
nutrient, 4, 5, 41

O

ocular vesicle, 1, 2, 5
old age, 2
opacification, 63, 65, 71
opacity, xii, xiii, 13, 14, 15, 16, 17, 31, 36, 39, 40, 41, 42, 45, 47
optic nerve, 21
optical properties, 45
orbit, 60
organ, 6, 44, 67, 73
organelles, 3, 16, 32, 45
organism, 39, 45, 61, 64, 66, 72
oxidative stress, 64
oxygen, 11, 14, 63

P

parenchyma, 72
pathogenesis, vii, ix, xii, 12, 23, 25, 33, 40, 41, 43, 47, 61, 73
pathological aging, xiii, 36, 44, 47
pathology, xiii, 12, 16, 22, 24, 44, 61, 67, 72
peptide(s), 5, 59
periodicity, 14
permeability, 13, 24, 39, 43, 44
pH, 29
phenotype(s), xiii, 19, 20, 36, 44, 45, 47, 66
Physiological, 71
physiology, 18, 62, 75
plasticity, 19, 35, 36
PMMA, 65
polarity, 20
polymers, 23
polystyrene, 28
population, 62
potassium, 13
pregnancy, 74
preparation, 28
prevention, xi, 13, 43, 69
probability, 17
progesterone, 75
progesteronic, xii, 11, 42
prolapse, 19

proliferation, 4, 65, 69, 71
prophylaxis, 7, 39, 68
protection, 13, 18, 74
protein-protein interactions, 63
proteins, 3, 12, 14, 24, 45, 69

R

race, 17
radiation, 17, 75
radio, 66
radius, 10
reactions, xiii, 22, 28, 35, 44, 57, 61, 64, 66, 73
receptors, xii, 11, 12, 18, 21, 22, 24, 39, 42, 61, 64, 65, 70, 75
recommendations, 29
reconstruction, 41
redistribution, 23
regenerate, 5, 6
regeneration, vii, 2, 5, 6, 60, 72
rehabilitation, 63
reliability, 29
reparation, 5
repressor, 62
respiration, 14
response, 12, 22
restoration, 5, 6, 7, 15, 40
reticulum, 75
retina, 1, 3, 4, 5, 6, 11, 17, 21, 68
retinal detachment, 6, 19
rhythm, 59
risk, 11, 17, 18, 62
role of bioamines, xii
Russia, 65, 67, 72

S

safety, 67
scattering, 63, 64
scientific investigations, 19
sclera, 6, 12, 21, 49
sensitivity, 67

serotonin, 24, 25, 28, 33, 34, 35, 42, 43, 47, 53, 59, 63, 75
sex, xii, 11, 17, 18, 42, 65
sex hormones, xii, 11, 18, 42
sex steroid, 65
shape, 2, 6
showing, 36
signs, xi, 20, 31, 40, 45, 51, 52
silicon, 14
skin, 5, 66
smooth muscle, 67, 69
sodium, 12
solution, 28, 29
specialists, 70
specialization, 45
spleen, 64, 72
stability, xiii
state, xii, xiii, 13, 15, 18, 24, 34
statistical processing, 29
statistics, 64
stimulation, 12, 14, 22, 24, 59, 67
stimulus, 72
stress, 68
structural changes, 14, 25
structure, vii, 7, 32, 39, 45, 49, 53, 63, 65
substrate, 14, 29
sulfur, 13, 43
Sun, 75
supervision, 22, 64
surgical removal, 17
swelling, 15, 18, 23
syndrome, xi, 16, 66, 71
synthesis, 2, 5, 6, 23, 24, 69

T

techniques, 61
temperature, 27, 29
tension, 2, 9, 14
terminals, 65
texture, 63
TGF, 11, 19
therapy, 33

thymus, 64, 65, 68, 72
thyroid, 72, 74
tissue, xiii, 4, 24, 43, 65, 72, 75
trace elements, 13, 14
transduction, 20
transformation, 1, 3, 6, 19, 32, 36, 44, 45
transforming growth factor, 7, 11, 19, 20
transmission, 6, 16, 18, 41
transparency, xi, 7, 10, 14
transplantation, 5, 27
transport, 42, 63
treatment, xi, xii, 25, 27, 29, 39, 62, 67, 70
tyrosine, 15

U

Ukraine, 70
ultrastructure, 70
USA, 62
USSR, 61, 67, 69

V

vapor, 27
varieties, 6, 16, 19, 39
vesicle, 1, 2, 3, 4, 5, 68
vessels, 4, 9, 31
vision, 10, 28, 44, 67, 73, 74
visual acuity, xi, 31, 40
visualization, 29

W

water, 10, 14, 17, 28, 29, 31, 40
water vapor, 28

Z

zinc, 13